Educational Outcomes
for Students with Disabilities

Educational Outcomes for Students with Disabilities

James E. Ysseldyke
Martha L. Thurlow
Editors

The Haworth Press, Inc.
New York · London

Educational Outcomes for Students with Disabilities has also been published as *Special Services in the Schools*, Volume 9, Number 2 1994.

The development, preparation, and publication of this work has been undertaken with great care. However, the publisher, employees, editors, and agents of The Haworth Press and all imprints of The Haworth Press, Inc., including The Haworth Medical Press and Pharmaceutical Products Press, are not responsible for any errors contained herein or for consequences that may ensue from use of materials or information contained in this work. Opinions expressed by the author(s) are not necessarily those of The Haworth Press, Inc.

The Haworth Press, Inc., 10 Alice Street, Binghamton, NY 13904-1580 USA

Library of Congress Cataloging-in-Publication Data

Educational outcomes for students with disabilities / James E. Ysseldyke, Martha L. Thurlow, editors.
     p. cm.
    Previously published in: Special services in the schools, v. 9, no. 2, 1994.
    Includes bibliographical references.
    ISBN 1-56024-743-6 (alk. paper)
    1. Handicapped children–Education–United States. 2. Educational tests and measurements–United States. 3. Educational evaluation–United States. 4. Education and state–United States. 5. Educational change–United States. I. Ysseldyke, James E. II. Thurlow, Martha L.
LC4031.E395 1995
371.91'0973–dc20
                                              95-11387
                                                CIP

AA2-9799

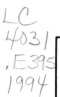
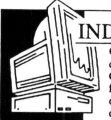

INDEXING & ABSTRACTING

Contributions to this publication are selectively indexed or abstracted in print, electronic, online, or CD-ROM version(s) of the reference tools and information services listed below. This list is current as of the copyright date of this publication. See the end of this section for additional notes.

- *Cabell's Directory of Publishing Opportunities in Education (comprehensive & descriptive bibliographic listing with editorial criteria and publication production data for selected education and education-related journals)*, Cabell Publishing Company, Box 5428, Tobe Hahn Station, Beaumont, TX 77726-5428

- *Child Development Abstracts & Bibliography*, University of Kansas, 2 Bailey Hall, Lawrence, KS 66045

- *Contents Pages in Education*, Carfax Information Systems, P.O. Box 25, Abingdon, Oxfordshire OX14 3UE, United Kingdom

- *Education Digest*, Prakken Publications, Inc., 416 Longshore Drive/P.O. Box 8623, Ann Arbor, MI 48107

- *Educational Administration Abstracts (EAA)*, Sage Publications, Inc., 2455 Teller Road, Newbury Park, CA 91320

- *ERIC Clearinghouse on Counseling and Student Services (ERIC/CASS)*, University of North Carolina-Greensboro, 101 Park Building, Greensboro, NC 27412-5001

- *ERIC Clearinghouse on Rural Education & Small Schools*, Appalachia Educational Laboratory, 1031 Quarrier Street, P.O. Box 1348, Charleston, WV 25325

(continued)

- *Exceptional Child Education Resources (ECER), (online through DIALOG and hard copy)*, The Council for Exceptional Children, 1920 Association Drive, Reston,VA 22091

- *International Bulletin of Bibliography on Education*, Proyecto B.I.B.E./Apartado 52, San Lorenzo del Escorial, Madrid, Spain

- *Inventory of Marriage and Family Literature (online and hard copy)*, National Council on Family Relations, 3989 Central Avenue NE, Suite 550, Minneapolis, MN 55421

- *Mental Health Abstracts (online through DIALOG)*, IFI/Plenum Data Company, 3202 Kirkwood Highway, Wilmington, DE 19808

- *National Clearinghouse for Bilingual Education*, George Washington University, 1118 22nd Street NW, Washington, DC 20037

- *OT BibSys*, American Occupational Therapy Foundation, P.O. Box 1725, Rockville, MD 20849-1725

- *Psychological Abstracts (PsycINFO)*, American Psychological Association, P.O. Box 91600, Washington, DC 20090-1600

- *Social Work Abstracts*, National Association of Social Workers, 750 First Street NW, 8th Floor, Washington, DC 20002

- *Sociology of Education Abstracts*, Carfax Publishing Company, P.O. Box 25, Abingdon, Oxfordshire OX14 3UE, United Kingdom

- *Special Educational Needs Abstracts*, Carfax Information Systems, P.O. Box 25, Abingdon, Oxfordshire OX14 3UE, United Kingdom

- *Urban Affairs Abstracts*, National League of Cities, 1301 Pennsylvania Avenue NW, Washington, DC 20004

(continued)

SPECIAL BIBLIOGRAPHIC NOTES

related to special journal issues (separates)
and indexing/abstracting

☐ indexing/abstracting services in this list will also cover material in any "separate" that is co-published simultaneously with Haworth's special thematic journal issue or DocuSerial. Indexing/abstracting usually covers material at the article/chapter level.

☐ monographic co-editions are intended for either non-subscribers or libraries which intend to purchase a second copy for their circulating collections.

☐ monographic co-editions are reported to all jobbers/wholesalers/approval plans. The source journal is listed as the "series" to assist the prevention of duplicate purchasing in the same manner utilized for books-in-series.

☐ to facilitate user/access services all indexing/abstracting services are encouraged to utilize the co-indexing entry note indicated at the bottom of the first page of each article/chapter/contribution.

☐ this is intended to assist a library user of any reference tool (whether print, electronic, online, or CD-ROM) to locate the monographic version if the library has purchased this version but not a subscription to the source journal.

☐ individual articles/chapters in any Haworth publication are also available through the Haworth Document Delivery Services (HDDS).

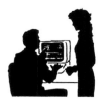

ABOUT THE EDITORS

James E. Ysseldyke, PhD, is Director of the National Center on Education Outcomes at the University of Minnesota in Minneapolis, where he is also Professor of Educational Psychology. He has been Principal Investigator for several studies funded by the U.S. Department of Education and has published a variety of articles on topics related to teaching and learning in special education.

Martha L. Thurlow, PhD, is Assistant Director of the National Center on Education Outcomes at the University of Minnesota in Minneapolis. She is the co-author of two books and over 75 book chapters and journal articles, as well as more than 100 reports from federally funded projects. Dr. Thurlow has also presented at 50 international, national, regional, state, and local conferences.

Educational Outcomes for Students with Disabilities

CONTENTS

Preface

Until very recently, school personnel usually responded to questions about the nature of special education with "process" or compliance responses: "We educate 437 students with disabilities," "We employ 37 resource teachers," "We have 4 self-contained classes," and "We have all of our students with disabilities on IEPs and re-evaluate them every three years." The scene has shifted. Process responses are no longer adequate in a time when legislators, bureaucrats and the general public are asking outcomes questions. The questions being asked, indeed the questions we must quickly address, sound like this: "How many of the students with disabilities who complete school in your system are literate?" "How many are physically fit?" and "How many have the necessary job skills to obtain and maintain gainful employment?"

This is a text about the results of education for students with disabilities. A number of issues and questions are addressed. What outcomes should we expect from educating students with disabilities? How should these outcomes be measured and reported? What do outcomes have to do with educational reform? What is Outcomes Based Education, what is outcomes-based accountability, and how do these two differ? What are opportunity-to-learn standards and what are the alternative ways of making judgments about whether students with disabilities get adequate opportunities to learn? How can national data collection programs contribute information that local educators can use to make policy decisions and improve outcomes for students in their districts? These are among the questions addressed in this book.

The term "outcomes" is a sensitive term among educators, one that is much used, much misused, and much maligned. In the first

[Haworth indexing entry note]: "Preface." Ysseldyke, James E., and Martha L. Thurlow. Published in *Educational Outcomes for Students with Disabilities* (ed: James E. Ysseldyke, and Martha Thurlow) The Haworth Press, Inc., 1994, pp. xv-xviii. Multiple copies of this article/chapter may be purchased from The Haworth Document Delivery Center [1-800-3-HAWORTH; 9:00 a.m. - 5:00 p.m. (EST)].

xv

article of this text, James Ysseldyke and Martha Thurlow explore the ways in which the term "outcomes" is used. They examine alternative conceptions of outcomes and identify the connotations each carries with it. Louis Danielson and David Malouf describe the ways in which federal policy on educational reform has been and is being used to achieve better results for students with disabilities.

Documenting the extent to which education works for students with disabilities is not a new federal, state, or local activity. Educators have struggled long and hard with the task of demonstrating that the extra services delivered to students with disabilities result in improved outcomes for the students. Kenneth Olsen reviews 15 years of efforts to evaluate the effectiveness of education for students with disabilities.

It is one thing to argue that we ought to document educational outcomes for students, and quite another to reach agreement on what ought to be measured. In article four, James Ysseldyke and Martha Thurlow describe the work of the National Center on Educational Outcomes in reaching national agreement on a conceptual model of educational outcomes and indicators.

In article five, Kevin McGrew describes the major national outcomes data collection activities, like the National Assessment of Educational Progress, and illustrates ways in which the data obtained through these large scale assessments can be used at the local level.

There are many forms of school reform legislation. One part of Goals 2000: The Educate America Act (PL 103-227) is a specification of voluntary opportunity to learn standards. What is opportunity to learn, how is it being defined in the professional literature, and what are the alternative ways in which it might be measured? Most importantly, what are the implications of opportunity to learn standards for students with disabilities? James Ysseldyke, Martha Thurlow, and Hyeonsook Shin address these questions in article six.

One cannot talk about outcomes or outcomes-based accountability without differentiating it from outcome-based education. Carol Massanari describes OBE and talks about what it means for students with disabilities. In article eight, LaMonte Wyche, Bob Algozzine and Michael Vanderwood describe an effort in the Washington, DC schools to use the NCEO model of outcomes and indicators to develop accountability measures for students with disabilities. In article nine, Michael Vanderwood and Ron Erickson discuss the consensus-building process that was used to develop the NCEO conceptual model. Martha Thurlow, James Ysseldyke, Michael Vanderwood and Gail Spande describe a Self-Study Guide to be used by school districts and states in developing systems of outcomes and indicators.

In article eleven, Elizabeth (Bette) Hyde describes ways in which related services personnel can contribute to school reform efforts and, in the twelfth article, James Shriner describes the debate about going beyond academics in accounting for educational outcomes.

In article thirteen, Cheryl Lange and James Ysseldyke report on outcomes of second chance programs like alternative schools and area learning centers.

In article fourteen, Cheri Gilman examines the reactions of administrators, teachers, and parents to the NCEO early childhood outcomes and indicators.

Alternative perspectives on identifying outcomes and setting standards are also presented. Nancy Verderber shares a personal perspective in which she emphasizes the need to consider the perspectives of people with disabilities when thinking about outcomes. Ann Turnbull and Janet Vohs provide a parent perspective on outcomes and indicators, discussing the risks of developing a system of outcomes and indicators that mention normal development and age appropriateness, and emphasizing the need to include parents in the process of model development.

Educational Outcomes for Students with Disabilities concludes with an article by Martha Thurlow, James Ysseldyke, and Kristin Geenen. In their look at future directions in educating students with disabilities, they identify four areas where there will be many emerging issues–implementation of Goals 2000, opportunity-to-learn standards, assessment accommodations, and accountability.

The development of this book was possible because the authors were willing to adhere to very short timelines. Completion of the total volume would still have been impossible without the many hours of reading and editing spent by Kristin Geenen and Rod Schaffer, both Graduate Research Assistants at the National Center on Educational Outcomes at the University of Minnesota. Furthermore, Kristin took upon and was successful in coordinating all communications with authors. And, of course, we want to thank Sheila Schedin, our word processor and secretary, for her great work in getting all articles in the same format, and making all final editing changes.

James E. Ysseldyke
Martha L. Thurlow
National Center on Educational Outcomes
University of Minnesota

Outcomes:
Watch Your Language!

James E. Ysseldyke
Martha L. Thurlow

National Center on Educational Outcomes
University of Minnesota

SUMMARY. The term "outcomes" today carries a lot of baggage with it. The term can mean many different things, but currently it has become a risky term to use. In this article, we describe why it is important for those who are interested in the education of students, and particularly the *results* of education for students with disabilities, to be careful in the language they use. We clarify the primary ways in which the word "outcomes" is used today–in outcome-based assessment, accountability, and education–and discuss why we must be careful in selecting our words.

Let's talk turkey.	*What's troubling you?*
Let's talk, Turkey.	*What's wrong with you?*

The *language* you use is important. And, *how* you use language is important. We are learning this lesson again very quickly in using the word "outcomes" in schools today.

The development of this article was supported in part by a Cooperative Agreement (H159C00004) between the University of Minnesota and the U.S. Department of Education, Office of Special Education Programs. Points of view or opinions expressed in the article are not necessarily those of the department or offices within it.

Address correspondence to: James E. Ysseldyke, 350 Elliott Hall, 75 East River Road, University of Minnesota, Minneapolis, MN 55455.

[Haworth co-indexing entry note]: "Outcomes: Watch Your Language!" Ysseldyke, James E., and Martha L. Thurlow. Co-published simultaneously in *Special Services in the Schools* (The Haworth Press, Inc.) Vol. 9, No. 2, 1994, pp. 1-10; and: *Educational Outcomes for Students with Disabilities* (ed: James E. Ysseldyke, and Martha L. Thurlow) The Haworth Press, Inc., 1994, pp. 1-10. Multiple copies of this article/chapter may be purchased from The Haworth Document Delivery Center [1-800-3-HAWORTH; 9:00 a.m. - 5:00 p.m. (EST)].

In this special volume, we are focusing on educational outcomes for students with disabilities. As you begin to read the many perspectives on outcomes presented in this special volume, you will need to understand what we mean when we say "outcomes." At least three different terms, formed by conjoining "outcomes" with other words, need to be defined: outcome-based assessment, outcome-based accountability, and outcome-based education. Before we discuss these additional terms, we provide examples of how the term "outcomes" is being used today. We conclude with evidence of why we need to be careful about how we use the word "outcomes."

DICTIONARY DEFINITIONS

The term "outcome" is defined in Webster's Ninth New Collegiate Dictionary (1988) as "something that follows as a result or consequence." It presents the word "effect" as a synonym for "outcome." The word "effect," in turn, is defined as "something that inevitably follows an antecedent (as a cause or agent); outcome is the final result of complex or conflicting causes or forces."

The National Center on Educational Outcomes (Ysseldyke, Thurlow, Bruininks, Deno, McGrew, & Shriner, 1991) defined the term to mean "the result of interactions between individuals and schooling experiences" (p. 8). Many times, the term has been defined by differentiating it from related terms, most often the "process" of education. Chester Finn (1990), former secretary of education, was one of many individuals who noted the contrast between the *process* of education and the *results* of education. He emphasized the need for a shift from a focus on the process of education (student-teacher ratio, number of library books, etc.) to a focus on the results of education (knowledge and skills of students). This kind of shift is now underway.

There are many reasons for the shift in focus, most of which reflect disappointment about what students who graduate from school know and are able to do. Businesses have expressed concern about the lack of work skills of students who graduate from school (Committee for Economic Development, 1991; Secretary's Commission on Achieving Necessary Skills, 1991). In international comparisons, the academic performance of United States students was near the bottom (Centre for Educational Research and Innovation, 1992; Elley, 1992; McKnight, Crosswhite, Dossey, Kifer, Swafford, Travers, & Cooney, 1989). Furthermore, the percentage of students actually completing high school in the United States is still relatively low, at approximately 75% to 85% nationwide (National Education Goals Panel, 1993; Office of Educational Research and Improvement, 1993), and the graduation rate even lower. The combination of too many students failing to graduate and concerns about the knowledge and skills of those who did graduate indicated to policymakers that unless something is changed, very soon the United States will be unable to compete in the global economy.

Our nation's governors and presidents (Bush and Clinton) have embraced the notion of educational outcomes in the form of national education goals. Starting with the six goals delineated by Bush and the governors, the National Governors' Association (1990) stated that: "Learning outcomes should reflect the skills, knowledge, and attitudes students need to prepare them for employment, further education, and responsible citizenship" (p. 17). Two goals were added to the original six during the legislative process to put into law *Goals 2000*, which codified the goals and the notion of educational reform though federally supported state reforms. The added goals, Goal 4 and Goal 8 (see Table 1), focused on the process variables of parent involvement and teacher training. Still, the education reform legislation emphasizes the importance of outcomes and measuring progress toward them.

HOW THE TERM "OUTCOMES" IS BEING USED

Since 1990, the term "outcomes" has appeared in educational literature with considerable frequency. In an ERIC search of documents published between 1990 and 1993, the term "outcomes" appeared in the title or abstract 272 times. Most of the time (43.0%), the term was used without modification, or with a general descriptor such as "educational," "learning," "positive," or "student" (30.1%). The following are some of the other words used to modify the term "outcomes":

academic	employment	program/project
achievement	family	social
affective	functional	transition
behavior(al)	graduation	treatment
career	high performance	vocational
development	language	work based

With one exception, the modifier was positioned *before* the word "outcomes" (e.g., family outcomes, transition outcomes, work-based outcomes). The one exception was the phrase "outcome-based education," which occurred approximately 3.3% of the time.

"OUTCOMES" WITH ASSESSMENT, ACCOUNTABILITY, AND EDUCATION

The term "outcome-based education" has produced the most controversy and is the reason you need to watch your language. It is, therefore, important to distinguish between this term and other terms like "outcome-based assessment" and "outcome-based accountability." Yet, even if you do understand the distinctions, be wary of those who treat any term that includes the word "outcome" as objectionable.

Outcome-based assessment is the term used to indicate that an assessment is based on, or designed to assess, specific pre-defined results. The desired outcomes for such assessments are higher-order kinds of skills rather than repetition of facts. Higher-order skills include reasoning, problem solving, and synthesizing knowledge. Today, outcome-based assessment generally implies that the assessment is of a new form as well. Most commonly referred to as "performance assessment" or "authentic assessment," the new form of assessment is assumed to better match the new kinds of outcomes that are being assessed. The use of such assessments is no longer limited to the classroom. Instead, performance assessments are being touted as a new tool of accountability and as needed even in large-scale assessment programs at the state level (Thurlow, 1994).

Outcome-based accountability refers to the use of performance on outcomes as the means to hold the school, or the school district, or the state, accountable for providing an education that produces

TABLE 1. National Education Goals

1. *School Readiness.* By the year 2000, all children in America will start school ready to learn.
2. *School Completion.* By the year 2000, the high school graduation rate will increase to at least 90 percent.
3. *Student Achievement and Citizenship.* By the year 2000, all students will leave grades 4, 8, and 12 having demonstrated competency over challenging subject matter including English, mathematics, science, foreign languages, civics and government, economics, arts, history, and geography, and every school in America will ensure that all students learn to use their minds well, so they may be prepared for responsible citizenship, further learning, and productive employment in our Nation's modern economy.
4. *Teacher Education and Professional Development.* By the year 2000, the Nation's teaching force will have access to programs for the continued improvement of their professional skills and the opportunity to acquire the knowledge and skills needed to instruct and prepare all American students for the next century.
5. *Mathematics and Science.* By the year 2000, United States students will be first in the world in mathematics and science achievement.
6. *Adult Literacy and Lifelong Learning.* By the year 2000, every adult American will be literate and will possess the knowledge and skills necessary to compete in a global economy and exercise the rights and responsibilities of citizenship.
7. *Safe, Disciplined, and Alcohol- and Drug-Free Schools.* By the year 2000, every school in the United States will be free of drugs, violence, and the unauthorized presence of firearms and alcohol and will offer a disciplined environment conducive to learning.
8. *Parental Participation.* By the year 2000, every school will promote partnerships that will increase parental involvement and participation in promoting the social, emotional, and academic growth of children.

specific desired outcomes. With the term accountability comes the notion that there are consequences for either reaching or not reaching the desired outcomes. Rewards and sanctions are the tools of consequence. The Center for Policy Options in Special Education (1994) identified two basic approaches to consequences: (a) rewards and sanctions based on incentive systems, and (b) public disclosure systems. Rewards and sanctions based on incentives may include monetary awards or losses to schools, the assignment of corrective action status and technical assistance to poorly performing schools, the use of waivers and regulatory flexibility, school or district closures or takeovers, monetary awards to teachers, graduation and postschool opportunities tied to school performance. Rewards and sanctions based on public disclosure systems include school or district level report cards and parental choice of school or districts. Accountability is a "systematic method to assure those inside and outside the educational system that schools and students are moving toward desired goals" (Center for Policy Options, 1994, p. 2).

Outcome-based education (OBE) is the term that has generated most of the concern about using the word "outcome." Original use and definition of this term came from William Spady, who argued for the need for education to be outcome-based, with direct linkages among outcomes, instruction, and assessment (see Spady & Marshall, 1991). The original conception was that given an outcome, some students would take more time to reach it than others. Thus, instruction should disregard the regular school calendar, and instead should be designed so that all students reach desired outcomes. This would mean that some students would require more time than others, and therefore, should not be bound by the calendar or by school schedules.

Spady's notion of a curriculum that is driven by outcomes depended on the setting of meaningful outcomes. Spady argued that such outcomes were not bound by content area, but rather reflected the integration of content and process knowledge. Typically, Spady-type outcomes were similar to the following:

- The student will be a self-directed learner
- The student will be a collaborative worker
- The student will be a complex thinker
- The student will be a community contributor
- The student will be a quality producer

It was these types of outcomes that got OBE into trouble with certain groups that believed the role of schools should be only to enhance academic achievement, not to teach values or behavior (see also, the article by Shriner in this volume).

OBE TROUBLE

The "trouble" started first in the form of objections in public meetings. Probably the first incident like this took place in Pennsylvania, where state leaders had decided to develop an educational system directed toward and evaluated in terms of the achievement of outcomes (Harp, 1993). Soon the objections were occurring not just in public meetings, but also in letters to the editor. An entire issue of *Educational Leadership* was devoted to the topic of "Can Public Schools Accommodate Christian Fundamentalists?" (December 1993/January 1994, Vol. 51, No. 4), with articles on OBE in Pennsylvania (McQuaide & Pliska, 1993-94) and the question "To Be or Not to OBE" (Ledell, 1993-94) among the articles. Below is an excerpt from one emotional letter sent by Dick Armey, a member of Congress, to his colleagues:

> OBE is real. It's bad. And it produces angry parents. . . . Just what is OBE? Boil away all the rhetoric about "world class standards," etc. . . . It holds smart children back to the pace of the slowest learners. . . . Soon, children are taking tests with open-ended questions like "Three things I don't like about my parents are . . ." . . . if you want those angry phone calls multiplied by 100, go right ahead, vote for OBE.

Individuals with conservative, anti-OBE views were being elected to local school boards. As this was accomplished, school districts that had signed on to the Spady notion of OBE began to have school boards that were opposing and overturning outcome-based systems (Richardson, 1994). Electronic mail in our own city carried the headline "ALL THE PEOPLE CANNOT BE FOOLED ALL THE TIME: OBE BY ANY OTHER NAME IS STILL SATANIC BRAINWASHING OF CHILDREN" and had choice phrases such as: "The parents of Minnesota will not allow our children's minds to be raped by spiritual child molesters. To find out what you can do, contact . . ."

Objections to OBE, and even to the term "outcomes" continued to increase, to the point where entire reports were being revised to contain words like "results" and "products" rather than "outcomes." A recent issue of *News & Views* (February, 1994, Vol. XIII,

No. 2), which presents selected articles to highlight key education issues, included nine articles supposedly related to OBE. The articles are listed in Table 2.

WHY WE MUST BE CAREFUL WHEN WE USE THE TERM "OUTCOMES"

It is clear from the above words, that we must be careful when we use the term "outcomes." Often the word is misinterpreted, but the

TABLE 2. A Sampling of Articles on OBE

Outcome-Based Education. Summary of Remarks by William J. Bennett, May 27, 1993. *Empower America.*

Do You Know Your Education Jargon? *The News-Sentinel*, July 26-31, 1993.

"Outcomes-Based" Education: An Overview. Education Commission of the States, 1993.

Dumbing Down Our Kids: What's Really Wrong with Outcome-Based Education, by Charles J. Sykes. *Wisconsin Interest.*

Outcome-Based Education by Robert G. Holland. *Chronicles*, September, 1993.

What Does It Mean to Focus on Education Outcomes? by Bruno V. Manno.

Hushed Takeover of American Education. *The Washington Times,* October 25, 1993.

Parent Power by James A. Barnes. *National Journal,* June 12, 1993.

Mastery Learning Reconsidered by Robert E. Slavin. *Review of Educational Research,* Summer 1987.

Note: These articles appeared in *News & Views* (February 1994, Vol. XIII, No. 2). The citation is based on all information that was included in the *News & Views* issue. It should be noted, however, that to the last article was the following disclaimer from Slavin: "I'm writing in response to your inquiry about a review I wrote in 1987 that is being used by opponents of Outcomes Based Education (OBE) all over the country. This review, published in the *Review of Educational Research,* involved group-based mastery learning, which has little in common with OBE. Use of my review as evidence against OBE is totally irresponsible and inappropriate. I wish I could find a way to stop opponents of OBE from using my research out of context, and hope this letter will serve that purpose" (Dated September 29, 1993).

concept behind the term is one that intertwines all the articles in this volume. We are concerned with how special services personnel understand the need to begin to focus on the *results* of education, not just the *process* of education. We believe that special services providers can be leaders in a move toward educational accountability for all students regardless of how at risk they may be, or of the disabilities they have.

We must be very clear when we talk about outcomes. The term "outcomes" is a discriminative stimulus for very many beliefs, thoughts, and perspectives. In short, the term carries much "excess baggage." We regularly encourage educators to use those synonyms of "outcomes" (e.g., results, values, products) they mean when they use the term. And, when the term is used, it is wise to state precisely how it is used. It is probably helpful to remember the words of Alice as she conversed with Humpty in *Through the Looking Glass:*

"I don't know what you mean by 'glory,'" Alice said.

Humpty Dumpty smiled contemptuously. "Of course you don't–till I tell you. I meant 'there's a nice knock-down argument for you!'"

"But glory doesn't mean 'a nice knockdown argument,'" Alice objected.

"When I use a word," Humpty Dumpty said, in rather a scornful tone, "it means just what I choose it to mean–neither more nor less."

"The question is," said Alice, "whether you *can* make words mean so many different things."

"The question is," said Humpty Dumpty, "which is to be master–that's all."

(Carroll, 1982, p. 136)

REFERENCES

Carroll, L. (1982). *The complete illustrated works of Lewis Carroll.* City: Crown.
Center for Policy Options in Special Education. (1994). *Issues & options in outcomes-based accountability for students with disability.* College Park, MD: University of Maryland.

Centre for Educational Research and Innovation. (1992). *Education at a glance: OECD indicators.* Paris, France: Organisation for Economic Cooperation and Development.

Committee for Economic Development. (1991). *The unfinished agenda: A new vision for child development and education.* Washington, DC: Author.

Elley, W. B. (1992). *How in the world do students read?* Hamburg, Germany: International Association for the Evaluation of Educational Achievement.

Finn, C. E. (1990). The biggest reform of all. *Phi Delta Kappan, 71*, 584-592.

Harp, L. (1993, September 22). Pa. parent becomes mother of 'outcomes' revolt. *Education Week, 13*(3), 1, 19-21.

Ledell, M. A. (1993-94). To be or not to OBE. *Educational Leadership, 51*(4), 18-19.

McKnight, C. C., Crosswhite, F. J., Dossey, J. A., Kifer, E., Swafford, J. O., Travers, K. J., & Cooney, T. J. (1990). *The underachieving curriculum: Assessing U.S. school mathematics from an international perspective. A national report on the Second International Mathematics Study.* Champaign, IL: Stipes Publishing.

McQuaide, J., & Pliska, A. (1993-94). The challenge to Pennsylvania's education reform. *Educational Leadership, 51*(4), 16-20.

National Education Goals Panel. (1993). *The national education goals report 1993. Vol 1: The National Report.* Washington, DC: U.S. Government Printing Office.

National Governors' Association. (1990). *National goals for education.* Washington, DC: Author.

Office of Educational Research and Improvement. (1993). *Reaching the goals: Goal 2–High school completion.* Washington, DC: U.S. Department of Education, Goal 2 Work Group.

Richardson, J. (1994, June 1). Minn. district scraps O.B.E. experiment seen as a model. *Education Week, 13*(36), 3.

Secretary's Commission on Achieving Necessary Skills. (1991, June). *What work requires of schools: A SCANS report for America 2000.* Washington, DC: U.S. Department of Labor.

Spady, W. G., & Marshall, K. J. (1991). Beyond traditional outcome-based education. *Educational Leadership, 49* (2), 73-75.

Thurlow, M. L. (1994). *National and state perspectives on performance assessment and students with disabilities* (CEC Mini-Library on Performance Assessment). Reston, VA: Council for Exceptional Children.

Ysseldyke, J. E., Thurlow, M. L., Bruininks, R. H., Deno, S. L., McGrew, K. S., & Shriner, J. G. (1991). *A conceptual model of educational outcomes for children and youth with disabilities* (Working Paper 1). Minneapolis, MN: National Center on Educational Outcomes, University of Minnesota.

Federal Policy and Educational Ret
Achieving Better Outcomes
for Students with Disabilities

Louis C. Danielson
David B. Malouf

Division of Innovation and Development
Office of Special Education Programs
Office of Special Education and Rehabilitative Services
U.S. Department of Education

SUMMARY. Substantial progress has been made during the past 20 years in the implementation of the original statute to provide educational services to students with disabilities (Public Law 94-142). Current concerns focus on opinions and data that indicate that implementation of the procedural requirements of the law has not led to satisfactory outcomes for students with disabilities. The possible role of the Goals 2000: Educate America Act in promoting better outcomes for students with disabilities, and other federal policy options for achieving better educational outcomes, are discussed.

A previous version of this article was presented as a paper by the first author at the Anglo-American Symposium on School Reform and Special Educational Needs in Cambridge, England, July, 1994. The opinions expressed in this article are those of the authors and do not necessarily reflect the position or policy of the U.S. Department of Education; official endorsement is neither implied, nor should it be inferred.

Address correspondence to: Louis C. Danielson, OSEP, 400 Maryland Avenue, SW, Capitol MES RM 3532, Washington, DC 20202.

[Haworth co-indexing entry note]: "Federal Policy and Educational Reform: Achieving Better Outcomes for Students with Disabilities." Danielson, Louis C., and David B. Malouf. Co-published simultaneously in *Special Services in the Schools* (The Haworth Press, Inc.) Vol. 9, No. 2, 1994, pp. 11-19; and: *Educational Outcomes for Students with Disabilities* (ed: James E. Ysseldyke, and Martha L. Thurlow) The Haworth Press, Inc., 1994, pp. 11-19. Multiple copies of this article/chapter may be purchased from The Haworth Document Delivery Center [1-800-3-HAWORTH; 9:00 a.m. - 5:00 p.m. (EST)].

11

12   ED¹ United States Congress enacted the Education for
In ᵉd Children Act (PL 94-142) to end the widespread
All children with disabilities from public schools and to
exᶜovision of appropriate services to the millions of stu-
eᵣ disabilities already in schools. The statute, currently
ₑ Individuals with Disabilities Education Act (IDEA),
plementing regulations provide very specific procedural
ents for schools to follow to ensure that its fundamental
ns (e.g., "free appropriate public education," "individual-
ucation programs," "least restrictive environment," etc.) are
mplicit in these requirements is the expectation that their
mentation will produce satisfactory educational outcomes for
ents with disabilities.

Over the years since enactment of the legislation, the federal
vernment has developed a comprehensive system for monitoring
ates' compliance with the provisions of the statute. States have
imilarly developed extensive systems to monitor the compliance of
local school districts. For the most part, compliance monitoring at
both the federal and state level has focused on the procedural
requirements of the law rather than the extent to which students
with disabilities achieve satisfactory outcomes.

Nearly 20 years have passed since the enactment of this land-
mark legislation, and the United States Congress is scheduled to
reauthorize the legislation. This is an opportune time to assess the
degree to which the goals of the legislation are being achieved and,
if not, to consider why not. While federal monitoring of states
continues to identify deficiencies in their programs, the overall
degree of implementation of the statute is substantial. No longer are
students with disabilities routinely excluded from schools. With few
exceptions, students have individualized education programs, and
parent notification and other procedural protections are provided. In
1975, the parents of a child with severe mental retardation typically
had the option of placing their child in an institution or keeping the
child at home. Today, that is unimaginable. In 1975, a student with
serious emotional disturbance would very likely be expelled from
school. Today, that is unlikely to happen, but if it does, the procedural protections of the statute provide a mechanism to challenge
the decision.

While substantial progress has been made, a concern has recently arisen that the implementation of procedural requirements has not led to satisfactory outcomes for students with disabilities. Until recently, no federal data were even collected to assess the adequacy of these educational outcomes. Perhaps we were preoccupied with process, confident in the process, or fearful of considering the outcomes. In the mid-1980s, Congress mandated a longitudinal study that would report on the secondary school experiences of a sample of students with disabilities and also assess post-secondary outcomes in employment, independent living, and education. Over the past three years, the data from this major study have become available and have provided a wake-up call for all concerned with the education of students with disabilities. Some of the most significant findings for youth with disabilities were reported by Wagner, Newman, D'Amigo, Jay, Butler-Nalin, Marder, and Cox (1991), who found that within two years of leaving school:

- Only 15% had attended a postsecondary school in the preceding year
- 30% had not held a paid job
- 40% of those employed had only worked part time
- 1 in 5 overall had been arrested
- 1 in 3 students with serious emotional disturbance had been arrested
- nearly 40% of youth left school by dropping out

The overall conclusion from these data is that the current system is failing many students with disabilities. Since the focus on procedural compliance has apparently been insufficient for ensuring that students with disabilities achieve satisfactory outcomes, it can be argued that we need to expand our focus to include accountability for student outcomes. Such a shift would be consistent with the emphasis on accountability for results that has become a central element of general education reform strategies in the United States. The Goals 2000: Educate America Act (PL 103-227), enacted in March 1994, reflects the critical role of outcome accountability in school reform activities.

This article addresses several of the issues related to federal policy and reform. What will be the impact of Goals 2000 on students with disabilities? Will students with disabilities be included in the accountability system and reforms that result from Goals 2000? Given that the U.S. Department of Education intends to align other major federal legislation with Goals 2000, what will this mean for the reauthorization of IDEA? The answers to these questions will have a direct impact on the delivery of related and special services.

THE GOALS 2000: EDUCATE AMERICA ACT

The general purpose and provisions of the act. Goals 2000 is intended to stimulate and facilitate the development and implementation of comprehensive education reforms aimed at helping "all" students reach challenging educational standards. Goals 2000 provides for the establishment of a National Education Standards and Improvement Council (NESIC) to review and certify voluntary national content and performance standards that define what all students should be able to do; certify voluntary "opportunity to learn" standards that describe the conditions of teaching and learning necessary for all students to have a fair opportunity to achieve to the level of the standards; and certify state standards and assessments. Perhaps because of historical concerns about federal encroachment in state and local educational autonomy, much of the national review is conducted by independent groups and submission of state standards and assessments is voluntary.

In order to receive funding under Goals 2000 each state must develop a comprehensive improvement plan through a broad-based panel comprised of legislators, state board members, teachers, principals, parents, representatives of business, labor, and higher education, and other members of the public. In addition, the statute indicates that the panel should be representative of the state with regard to race, ethnicity, gender, and disability characteristics. The plans must address:

- Strategies for developing and adopting content and performance standards, student assessments, and plans for teacher training;
- Strategies for providing all students an opportunity to learn at higher academic levels;

- Strategies for improving management and governance, and for promoting accountability for results, flexibility, site-based management, and other principles of high-performance management;
- Strategies for involving parents and the community in helping all students meet the challenging state standards and for promoting grass-roots, bottom-up involvement in reform;
- Strategies for ensuring that all local educational agencies and schools in the state are involved in developing and implementing needed improvements; and
- Strategies for assisting local educational agencies and schools to meet the needs of school-aged students who have dropped out of school.

School districts in states receiving Goals 2000 funding must apply for funds on a competitive basis with a local improvement plan developed by a broad-based panel with diverse membership, including persons with disabilities. The bulk of the funds received by a local education agency must be made available to individual schools to develop and implement comprehensive school improvement plans designed to help all students achieve state content and performance standards.

Goals 2000 also authorizes states and school districts to obtain waivers from the requirements of several federal programs including the Chapter 1 program for disadvantaged students and the vocational education program. The state must demonstrate that the requirements to be waived are impeding their ability to execute their improvement plan. The Statute also provides for six state flexibility demonstration programs, which essentially exchange flexibility for accountability. States must also waive their state regulations under these provisions. The provisions of civil rights laws and those of IDEA are not among those that can be waived.

Another important provision of Goals 2000 is that funds may be used to improve preservice teacher education programs consistent with the state improvement plan and to support continuing professional development activities. These grants are to be made through a competitive, peer-reviewed process to local school districts or consortia of local districts, in cooperation with institutions of higher education or nonprofit organizations. Applications that target preparation and professional development for teachers of students with disabilities are among the priorities. It is interesting to note that these grants go to local districts and not institutions of higher education, although it seems clear that the districts are expected to work cooperatively with higher education.

Goals 2000 and students with disabilities. How does Goals 2000 apply to students with disabilities and what implications does the bill have for them? The term "all students" is defined to include students with disabilities, and the bill makes it clear that "all" students are to be included in the school reform activities that it authorizes. The Congressional report accompanying the bill contains several pages of discussion regarding the participation of students with disabilities in Goals 2000 activities, including the following language:

> The Committee intends that the exclusion of individuals with disabilities from any aspect of . . . reform is unacceptable. . . . [There is] an expectation that all students across a broad range of performance will be held to high standards if they are to realize their full potential. (U.S. Congress, 1993, p. 20)

In part because of concern that students with disabilities have not been explicitly considered in many school reform activities, Goals 2000 mandates a comprehensive study of the inclusion of children with disabilities in school reform activities assisted under the Act. Among the issues the study is required to address are:

1. An evaluation of the National Education Goals and objectives, curricular reforms, standards, and other activities intended to achieve the goals;
2. A review of assessments and measures used to gauge progress toward the goals and standards; and
3. An examination of incentives or assistance that might be provided to ensure the development of improvement plans that adequately address students with disabilities.

This study was to start September 1994 and is required to be completed within two years.

Students with disabilities and educational antecedents to Goals 2000. Many of the provisions of Goals 2000 build upon activities that are actually already well under way. For example, the development of national standards in all the core academic subjects is nearing completion. The National Assessment of Educational Progress (NAEP) is already in place and is regarded by many as the method to be used to gauge the success of school reform activities at the national level. Many states are well along on their own reform efforts, and most already have assessments in place.

To study the extent to which students with disabilities have been included in these reform activities, the U.S. Office of Special Education Programs (OSEP) established the National Center on Educational Outcomes (NCEO) in 1990. Among the findings are that nearly 50% of students with disabilities have been excluded from national assessments, and similar patterns of exclusion are prevalent in state-level assessments (NCEO, 1992). Central to this problem are technical and policy issues related to testing accommodations (Thurlow, Ysseldyke, & Silverstein, 1993), as well as inconsistent policies related to inclusion or exclusion of students in assessment programs.

With regard to educational standards, until recently little attention has been paid to students with disabilities in standards development activities. Standards have been linked to educational data sources that typically exclude students with disabilities; they have focused on core academic subjects to the neglect of social and life skills that are important to many students with disabilities; and their appropriateness and feasibility for students with disabilities have been questioned (Thurlow & Ysseldyke, 1993).

There are notable exceptions to these patterns of exclusion. For example, Kentucky includes all students in its assessment activities. Over 99 percent of Kentucky students are in the general state assessment. The remaining students, who are primarily those with severe cognitive impairments, participate in an alternative portfolio assessment. However, it should be recognized that the prevailing trend has been to exclude students with disabilities from key aspects of educational reform at federal and state levels, and that this trend may not be easily overcome.

FEDERAL POLICY OPTIONS
FOR ACHIEVING BETTER EDUCATIONAL OUTCOMES
FOR STUDENTS WITH DISABILITIES

IDEA is distinct among federal education laws in the extent to which it combines program authorities with substantial federal mandates, monitoring, and accountability. These features are entirely understandable given the entrenched patterns of educational exclusion and inappropriate services that prevailed when PL 94-142 was first enacted. However, because this legislation has improved access to appropriate services without achieving satisfactory educational outcomes for a large number of students with disabilities, it can be argued that the time has come for us to focus more intensively on outcomes. Our first impulse might be to expand the existing mechanism for federal monitoring and accountability to include educational outcomes as well as processes. However, a range of alternative policy instruments are available, and consideration should be given to which are most likely to yield the desired results.

The reforms being undertaken in the general educational system in this country are motivated by the same concerns about poor educational outcomes that have arisen in special education. However, these reforms, as embodied in Goals 2000, are not based on centralized, top-down mandates. Instead, they are based on a systemic approach to educational change characterized by restructuring, local autonomy, reduction in centralized control and "red tape," and encouragement and support for local innovation accompanied by local accountability for results (Smith & O'Day, 1991).

Should special education policy makers consider this reform strategy as a means for achieving better outcomes for students with disabilities? The legalistic, top-down approaches that currently shape special education policy and governance may be effective for establishing procedural safeguards and gaining general access to educational services. However, such approaches can also result in passive compliance; they tend to constrain rather than enable the work of educators; and they are therefore highly questionable as instruments for stimulating the meaningful changes in educational practice needed to improve outcomes for students with disabilities (Weatherley & Lipsky, 1977; Fuller, Noel, & Malouf, 1985; Smith, 1990).

As we consider the impact of federal laws such as Goals 2000 and IDEA on students with disabilities, and the critical need to achieve better educational outcomes for these students, it may be appropriate to call for federal policies that balance centralized regulation and accountability with decentralized reforms. Federal mandates and compliance mechanisms may be necessary to ensure continued access to appropriate services, including access to general educational reforms. At the same time, federal support for decentralized, flexible, locally-driven reforms may be needed to improve educational outcomes. A key, unanswered question is the degree to which these two contrasting strategies can coexist. Can "street-level bureaucrats" (Weatherley & Lipsky, 1977) contribute to local educational reform?

REFERENCES

Fuller, B., Noel, M. M., & Malouf, D. M. (1985). Polity and competence: Can the state change teachers' skills? *Educational Evaluation and Policy Analysis* 7(4), 343-353.

National Center on Educational Outcomes. (1992). *Including students with disabilities in national and state data collection programs*. (Brief Report #1). Minneapolis, MN: University of Minnesota, National Center on Educational Outcomes.

Smith, S. W. (1990). Individualized education programs (IEPs) in special education—From intent to acquiescence. *Exceptional Children, 57*(1), 6-14.

Smith, M. S., & O'Day, J. (1990). Systemic school reform. In S. Fuhrman & B. Malen (Eds.), *The politics of curriculum and testing* (pp. 233-267). Philadelphia: The Falmer Press.

Thurlow, M. L., & Ysseldyke, J. E. (1993). *Can "all" ever really mean "all" in defining and assessing student outcomes?* (Synthesis Report 5). Minneapolis, MN: University of Minnesota, National Center on Educational Outcomes.

Thurlow, M. L., Ysseldyke, J. E., & Silverstein, B. (1993). *Testing accommodations for students with disabilities: A review of literature*. (Synthesis Report 4). Minneapolis, MN: University of Minnesota, National Canter on Educational Outcomes.

U.S. Congress. (1993). Goals 2000: Educate America Act. (Report from the Senate Committee on Labor and Human Resources, July 13,1993). Washington, DC: Author.

Wagner, M., Newman, L., D'Amico, R., Jay, E. D., Butler-Nalin, P., Marder, C., & Cox, R. (1991). *Youth with disabilities: How are they doing? The first comprehensive report from the National Longitudinal Transition Study of Special Education Students*. Menlo Park, CA: SRI International.

Weatherley, R., & Lipsky, M. (1977). Street-level bureaucrats and institutional innovation: Implementing special-education reform. *Harvard Educational Review, 47*(2), 171-197.

Have We Made Progress in Fifteen Years of Evaluating the Effectiveness of Special Education Programs?

Kenneth Olsen

Mid-South Regional Resource Center
Interdisciplinary Human Development Institute
University of Kentucky

SUMMARY. Fifteen years of evaluating the effectiveness of special education programs point to certain patterns that are informative for those in current reform efforts. In this article, the progression from local to state and federal control, from program improvement to accountability, from evaluation of process to outcome and back, and from simple to complex models is highlighted. Also examined is the trend toward developing a system that includes all students instead of just those in special education, concluding with a set of recommendations for evaluators and school professionals.

The desire of special educators to move beyond compliance monitoring to evaluating the effectiveness of special education programs

This article was developed pursuant to cooperative agreement #H028A30008-94, CFDA 84.028A between the Mid-South Regional Resource Center, Interdisciplinary Human Development Institute, University of Kentucky and the Office of Special Education Programs, U.S. Department of Education. However, the opinions expressed herein do not necessarily reflect the position or policy of the U.S. Office of Special Education Programs and no endorsement by that office should be inferred.

Address correspondence to: Kenneth Olsen, Mid-South RRC, University of Kentucky, 114 Minerals Industries Building, Lexington, KY 40506-0051.

[Haworth co-indexing entry note]: "Have We Made Progress in Fifteen Years of Evaluating the Effectiveness of Special Education Programs?" Olsen, Kenneth. Co-published simultaneously in *Special Services in the Schools* (The Haworth Press, Inc.) Vol. 9, No. 2, 1994, pp. 21-37; and: *Educational Outcomes for Students with Disabilities* (ed: James E. Ysseldyke, and Martha L. Thurlow) The Haworth Press, Inc., 1994, pp. 21-37. Multiple copies of this article/chapter may be purchased from The Haworth Document Delivery Center [1-800-3-HAWORTH; 9:00 a.m. - 5:00 p.m. (EST)].

has been expressed for over 15 years (e.g., Olsen, 1979). Approaches to evaluating effectiveness have been put forth since shortly after the passage of the Education for All Handicapped Children Act. Efforts have been made to evaluate effectiveness despite the lack of consistent definition of terms; lack of consensus on a conceptual model to interrelate the inputs, processes and outcomes in special education programs; and most importantly, lack of agreement on what it means to have an effective special education program (Borich, 1977). While all of these concerns still remain today, a number of significant changes are taking place in the ways that evaluation of services to students with disabilities is viewed and is approached. The purpose of this article is to provide evaluators and school professionals with a context for their work, to help them understand how we have arrived at this point and, perhaps, what is on the horizon.

Five strands of change can be identified that have implications for the present and future of special education program evaluation:

From	To
Schools and districts as locus of control, with limited federal involvement.	State and federal structures driving evaluation with more active Federal involvement.
Evaluation for program improvement.	Evaluation for accountability.
Evaluation of inputs and processes.	Evaluation of outcomes and effects in the context of inputs and processes.
Simple models of inputs, processes and outputs.	More sophisticated conceptual models taking in a larger number of factors.
Student learning outcomes specific to special education.	Integration of outcomes in larger general education and human service frameworks.

LOCAL TO STATE AND FEDERAL CONTROL

While most of the efforts of the '70s and '80s focused on helping schools and local education agencies (LEAs) plan and conduct evaluation (Olsen, 1984, 1986), there now is an increasing tendency for evaluations at state and federal levels. State and federal support for special education program evaluation has reflected this change.

In the 1970s, the U.S. Office of Special Education funded the Evaluation Training Consortium at Western Michigan University and the University of Virginia. The project culminated with the publication of an evaluation reference tool for special educators (Brinkerhoff, Brethower, Hluchyj, & Nowakowski, 1983) that spawned a number of state resource documents and training events. Workbook-type manuals and team training events in the states of Florida, Maine, Missouri, Kansas, Nebraska, Maryland, Virginia, West Virginia and Utah have roots in that guide. Similarly, the Missouri Special Education Evaluation System (SEES) (Missouri Section of Special Education, 1985) led to the Utah SEES (Utah Consortium of Local Directors of Special Education, 1988). The intent of each was to provide step-by-step guidance to help LEAs plan and conduct their own evaluations.

In 1988 the Council of Administrators of Special Education (CASE) produced *Education Program Evaluation: An Overview* (McLaughlin, 1988), which drew from earlier efforts to provide a workbook-type approach for local evaluations. Use of the CASE document either in original or adapted form was driven by locally identified needs and designed by local stakeholders.

During this same era, other states were providing local systems with general handbooks on evaluating special education programs (e.g., California Office of Special Education, 1982; Illinois State Board of Education, 1982; Rhode Island Department of Education, 1984). Other states were providing their LEAs with specific forms, data collection procedures, and report formats (e.g., Massachusetts Division of Special Education, 1981; North Carolina Division for Exceptional Children, 1983). However, LEAs were given the option of using those tools or others that they chose. Some commercial materials on special education evaluation were produced (Maher & Bennett, 1984; Nance & Borich, 1986), but these, too, presented methods for LEAs to select components of their special education system and design evaluations for those components. In addition to providing materials, training and technical assistance, some states (e.g., Maryland) provided incentive funding for LEA-initiated self studies (Olsen, 1986). States, therefore, have provided support for LEA evaluations but historically have not required use of common formats and procedures. As discussed by DeStefano

(1990), the lack of evaluation standardization "exacerbates problems associated with cross-site aggregation of evaluation data" (p. 262).

An increasing number of states are developing special education outcome and indicator systems that cut across LEA lines (e.g., Michigan, New Jersey) and nearly all states now are considering ways to move some of their state resources from monitoring LEAs for compliance to monitoring them for effectiveness. Over half of the states are exploring results-based or outcome-based monitoring, either as an alternative or adjunct to their systems of monitoring for compliance with federal and state requirements.

Evaluating the effectiveness of special education and individualized education programs (IEPs) as required by IDEA has proceeded without federal direction. For example, there has always been a requirement in state IDEA plans for a section on how the state will conduct evaluation of special education program effectiveness and the effectiveness of IEPs. However, until very recently, federal involvement in special education evaluation has paralleled state approaches (i.e., supporting local option evaluations and allowing states maximum flexibility in interpreting federal requirements). The National Association of State Directors of Special Education (NASDSE) analyzed the evaluation components of state plans over time and found:

- An increase in the number of states that discuss compliance monitoring in the annual evaluation sections of the State Plan and Part B Performance Report.
- An increase in the number of states that describe a two-tiered approach to the annual evaluation requirement, whereby the LEAs have specific evaluation requirements and the state has specific monitoring requirements.
- An increase in the number of states that encourage LEA "self-study." This practice was described by different states as a pre-monitoring tool or an evaluation tool.
- An increase in the number of states that provide technical assistance to LEAs to help them evaluate their programs and procedures (Gonzalez, 1992).

Such plans were approved by OSEP, and therefore the federal government tacitly endorsed evaluation as something that was locally designed and driven. Attempts were made by OSEP and its contractors in 1985, 1987 and 1990 to produce clear criteria for these sections of the state plans, but each attempt failed to be approved as an official guideline for state evaluation systems.

Perhaps the most aggressive federal effort to date has been the State Agency Federal Evaluation Studies (SAFES) program, which evolved from a series of unrelated and unguided studies, to specific investigations. Each study is guided by a cooperative agreement between the U.S. Department of Education and a state agency to conduct an evaluation of special education programs and services. Through this program, states propose evaluation studies and the federal government provides funding and technical assistance for the state-designed efforts.

The funding of the National Longitudinal Transition Study (NLTS) (Wagner, 1990), the National Center on Educational Outcomes (NCEO) at the University of Minnesota, and Performance Assessment for Self-Sufficiency–Project PASS (Campeau, 1993) is evidence of an increased federal interest in more commonality in state and national evaluations of services to students with disabilities. These projects also lend themselves to national data collection.

Therefore, both state and national support for evaluation of services to students with disabilities appears to be moving toward centralized information collection and away from driven evaluations. Olsen and Massanari (1991) argued for a balanced approach that includes both data on services to students with disabilities and data on the effects of those services, a system for SEA self-evaluation, *and* support for LEA self-evaluations. It is likely that pressure toward more centralized evaluation functions will continue as the public continues to demand more data on overall costs and effects of services for students with disabilities.

FROM PROGRAM IMPROVEMENT TO ACCOUNTABILITY

Paralleling the increasing emphasis on centralized evaluation is a change in the purpose for which special education evaluations are conducted. The clearly defined purposes of the past are giving way to a new purpose–accountability. Horvath (1985) defined evaluation for program improvement as a management tool to identity specific components of the LEA special education program that need attention. He defined evaluation for accountability as a way to provide information to administrative, regulatory, oversight or funding authorities about the operations and effects of a program.

The change from program improvement to accountability as the primary purpose for special education program evaluation is consistent with trends in general education. Questions are being raised about whether special education services are resulting in expected changes and whether the effort is worth the results that are being achieved (Lewis, 1991; Zirkel, 1990).

"Outcome-based accountability" and "results-based monitoring" have become bywords. The *National Agenda for Achieving Better Results for Children and Youth with Disabilities* recommends that special educators "implement accountability systems that monitor program effectiveness, balancing process with results, and provide incentives for program improvement and sanctions for noncompliance" (COSMOS, 1994, p. 18). Stakeholders are demanding information on the extent to which expected results are being obtained, and that rewards and sanctions be established as contingencies for accomplishment of outcomes.

The potential negative effects of using incentives and sanctions in a rigorous accountability approach to program evaluation in special education have yet to be fully explored (Center for Policy Options in Special Education, 1992; Olsen, 1994). While the debate continues to escalate about the feasibility of using the same assessment systems for both program accountability and improvement purposes, policymakers are proceeding as if there will be few problems. However, it is becoming increasingly apparent that high stakes environments can lead to superficial adherence to standards, inappropriate placements, and restricted curricula and instruction (Center for Policy Options in Special Education, 1992; Fullan, 1991; Rogers, 1983).

FROM EVALUATION OF PROCESS
TO OUTCOMES AND BACK AGAIN

Evaluation of special education programs and services has historically focused on answering such input questions as "Are staff qualified?" "Are materials available?" and "Are facilities accessible?" or such process questions as "Were parents involved in the decision process?" "Does the student's program match the IEP?" and "Are students participating with their nondisabled peers?" However, the growing dissatisfaction with input and process as the intent of special education and the increasing demand for more information on outcomes is well documented (Borich & Nance, 1987; George, George, & Grosenick, 1990; Olsen, 1979; Vogelsberg, 1994). Now there is a new realization—that outcome data without information on the programs and services that led to those outcomes will leave the public with no basis for making decisions about needed changes (Ysseldyke, Thurlow, Bruininks, Gilman, Deno, McGrew, & Shriner, 1992).

OSEP's Annual Reports to Congress provide information on the numbers of students in special education, on the number of teachers available and needed, and on the extent to which students are in integrated placements. Until recently, they have provided very little information on the outcomes of those inputs and processes (DeStefano & Wagner, 1990). A few special projects, such as the NLTS (Wagner, 1990), have provided the nation with a limited picture of outcomes. In *Serving Handicapped Children,* the Robert Wood Johnson Foundation (1988) stated that the "emphasis on the availability and use of services should not obscure concerns about the quality of these services, concerns that cannot be addressed without substantially more information about children's progress over time" (p. 17). Likewise, the report of the National Council on Disability (1989) described the feelings of parents, educators and taxpayers in every locale:

> The time has come to ask the same questions for students with disabilities that we have been asking about students without disabilities:
>
> - Are they achieving?
> - Are they staying in school?
> - Are they prepared to enter the work force when they finish school?
> - Are they going on to participate in postsecondary education and training?
> - Are they prepared for adult life (p. 2)?

In response, the *National Agenda* (COSMOS, 1994) recommended that agencies define program results and functional learning outcomes for children and youth with disabilities, and develop indicators that focus on those results in collaboration with children and youth, families and community members. States such as Michigan, Delaware, and Kentucky have made concerted efforts to produce disaggregated data on the achievement levels of students with disabilities. The NCEO has worked with the leaders of the National Assessment of Educational Progress to increase the number of students with disabilities included in assessment, with the intent of increasing the pool of information available on outcomes and improving the comparability of results across states (Ysseldyke, Thurlow, McGrew, & Vanderwood, 1994).

However, a number of authors have pointed out that information on outcomes, especially negative outcomes, provides little information about what actions to take to improve those outcomes (Horvath, 1992; Olsen & Massanari, 1991; Ysseldyke et al., 1992). While information on outcomes is necessary, it is not sufficient. There is growing awareness that it is essential also to have information on the inputs and processes that lead to achievement of outcomes. The national emphasis on "opportunity-to-learn standards" in Goals 2000 is evidence that the pendulum is swinging back to the middle. Opportunity-to-learn standards have yet to be defined, but most likely will be drawn from the effective schools literature (Porter, 1993). Porter suggests that such standards can be used to explain outcomes.

Future efforts to evaluate educational programs and services for students with disabilities must recognize the need to gather information at all levels of implementation in order to understand what outcomes are not being achieved and what adjustments are needed to improve those outcomes. Stakeholders might want to advocate for folding key provisions into local and state opportunity-to-learn standards.

FROM SIMPLE TO COMPLEX CONCEPTUAL MODELS

Chen (1990) suggested that evaluation is most effective when it is informed by a conceptual model of the program being evaluated.

Models used to drive special education evaluation have evolved from simple input-process-output lists to complex models that take into consideration context factors and external influences to special education services. The earliest models tended to be based on lists of activities or inputs, resources or processes, and outcomes or results that were considered to reflect an effective program, without demonstrating interrelationships among the components or taking into account factors outside a narrow special education focus (e.g., Borich, 1977; Gable, 1982; Lieberman & McNeil, 1982; Maher & Bennett, 1983; Olsen, 1979).

More recently, models for services to students with disabilities have started to take into account a greater number of variables. The New Hampshire special education program improvement partnership (Lachat et al., 1986) incorporates a multi-level model and a wide range of indicators in the areas of: (a) student and program outcomes; (b) philosophy, policies and procedures; (c) resources and the school program; (d) instructional practices; (e) staff competencies, attitudes, and relationships; (f) parent participation; (g) school and classroom climate; and (h) leadership. West Virginia developed a similar multi-level model that defined inputs, processes and outcomes in 10 activity areas (e.g., parent and community support; school based assistance teams). Outcomes from each activity are shown to be inputs for other activities and the interrelationships among effectiveness indicators is shown graphically and in narrative form (Olsen & Turley, 1988).

DeStefano and Wagner (1990) indicated that a conceptual framework for outcome assessment in special education should encompass not only school programs and services and student outcomes, but also school contexts, individual/family/community characteristics, young adult outcomes and adult programs/services.

Education, especially education of students with disabilities, can no longer be viewed as a simple factory model of inputs, processes and outputs. Influences are vast. In the future, persons evaluating special education programs will have to build into their conceptual models an increasing number of factors as human services become more interagency in nature and as educational services to students with disabilities become increasingly embedded in services for all students.

EFFECTIVENESS INDICATORS
FOR SPECIAL EDUCATION
TO EFFECTIVENESS INDICATORS FOR ALL

Effectiveness indicators in special education have been changing to reflect the changing service delivery system. In the past, indicators described special education inputs, processes and outcomes in isolation. Now, they are increasingly being described as a part of indicators for all students and for society in general.

One of the earliest attempts to synthesize effectiveness indicators in special education was the work by the National Regional Resource Center (RRC) Panel on Indicators of Effectiveness in Special Education (1986). The RRC program conducted needs assessments in all SEAs and found that over 60% of the states wanted a tool that agencies could use to judge their own effectiveness. Because many redundant activities existed on locating indicators of effectiveness in special education, research articles and state-developed indicator lists were synthesized into a comprehensive list of effectiveness indicators. These were organized into seven categories (philosophy; policies and practices; resource allocation; staffing and leadership; parent participation and community involvement; instruction; and program and student outcomes).

There were hundreds of indicators in the first sections of this document, but only a few in the program and student outcome section. Still, the indicator lists were used as adjuncts to state evaluation systems in several states (e.g., Maryland, New Hampshire, Florida); West Virginia added new literature on pre-referral processes and reformatted the indicators into inputs, processes and outputs according to their model (Olsen & Turley, 1988). While the document was linked to general education effectiveness indicators, it had a clear special education focus.

A number of other indicator documents specific to special education were produced in the 80s and reported in the literature (e.g., Bickel & Bickel, 1986), in state reference guidelines (e.g., Florida, Kansas) and in local school district standards documents (e.g., Jefferson County Public Schools, 1988). Most addressed special education programs. A variety of indicator documents also were developed for early childhood programs (e.g., Iowa's Early Childhood Special Education Review), secondary transition programs (e.g., Hasazi, Hock, & Cravedi-Cheng, 1993), and for services to students with severe disabilities (e.g., Halvorsen & Sailor, 1989; Kleinert, Smith, & Hudson, 1990). As with other efforts, these documents focused on practices and resources rather than effects and outcomes for special education.

The national movement toward inclusion is leading to a different view of effectiveness indicators for educational services to students with disabilities. Documents by Gartner and Lipsky (1989) and Stainback and Stainback (1984) called for a unitary system of education and the melding of special education personnel into a supportive role in regular education environments. The National Association of State Directors of Special Education endorsed this concept. In addition, the *National Agenda* calls for "a unified educational system [that] will incorporate equitable standards and high expectations for all children and youth" (COSMOS, 1994, p. 3).

General educators also are calling for a more inclusionary system. The National Association of State Boards of Education endorsed such a system in *Winners All* (NASBE, 1992). Goals 2000 codifies the eight national education goals and establishes a National Education Standards and Improvement Council (NESIC). The House and Senate committee language for Goals 2000 makes it clear that Congress intends for the National Education Standards and Improvement Council to ensure that state and local standard setting and assessment activities provide for *all* children in relation to the same eight national education goals.

The most recent effort to produce a comprehensive outcome and indicator system reflects this inclusionary orientation. NCEO developed a conceptual model of outcomes and has produced outcomes and indicators at six levels (age 3, age 6, grade 4, grade 8, students exiting school, and post school) in the areas of presence/participation, accommodation/adaptation/compensation, independence/responsibility, physical/mental health, social/behavior skills, contributions/citizenship, literacy, and satisfaction (Ysseldyke, Thurlow, & Shriner, 1992). While the specific names and organization of the model has changed (see Ysseldyke & Thurlow, this volume), the entire model continues to be based on an assumption of an integrated system. In fact, the conceptual model and all indicator documents are designed to apply to all students (Ysseldyke et al., 1992). State personnel also are being very careful to avoid being seen as separatists, ensuring that functional curricula and unique special education goals are eliminated or at least cross-matched to the outcomes and indicators for all students.

The debate regarding whether effectiveness indicators, and especially outcomes for all students, can meet the needs of students with disabilities is not over. Michigan has been engaged in a massive effort to identify unique category-specific outcomes for students (e.g., visual impairment, learning disability). The logic for separate outcomes has to do with the purpose of special education services. Michigan perceives that:

> the task of *special education* is *to limit handicaps, to compensate for the disability* or limit the inability, to enable individuals to access the same knowledge as his (sic) nonhandicapped peers. To do this, special education attempts to discover what *special education accommodations* are necessary for students with an impairment to learn and achieve in education. (Frey, 1991, p. 6, emphasis in original)

There is concern that the uniqueness of special education and its mission to provide specially designed instruction to students with disabilities will be lost. This concern is shared by those who fear that high expectations and common goals will mean that all students will have to meet the same standards in the same way regardless of disability, without accommodations (Little, 1993). Similarly, the disability community at large continues to have concerns about achieving positive outcomes unique to individuals with disabilities throughout all supports and services including residential, vocational, social, and educational. For example, the recently published *Outcome Based Performance Measures* by the Accreditation Council on Services for People with Disabilities (1993) specifies 30 life role outcome measures specific to people with disabilities and 17 outcome measures for organizations that provide supports and services for persons with disabilities.

Developers of outcomes and effectiveness indicators must find ways to maintain a focus on what makes education effective for all students. Still, they must ensure the availability of outcomes and indicators that provide a vision of effective practice and a basis for gathering information about how to better meet the needs of students with disabilities. Educators must be prepared to respond to the expectations of advocates and professionals for positive life role outcomes. Specifying both generic and specific outcomes may be the only way to address both needs.

CONCLUSIONS

After fifteen years, the evaluation of educational services to students with disabilities still lacks clear definitions of terms. Debates about purposes, standards and procedures abound. Clear guidance from the federal level regarding requirements for evaluating effectiveness of IEPs is still lacking, but there is expanding interest in having common data to answer critical outcome questions. Unfortunately, the orientation at state and national levels seems to have shifted from a focus on program improvement to a focus on accountability without a full understanding of how evaluative information might be affected by a high stakes environment. Evaluation of outcomes for students with disabilities and evaluation of the effects of supports and services to individuals with disabilities are now viewed in the broader framework of conceptual models that includes context, input and process variables that affect those outcomes and effects.

The past 15 years of experiences in evaluating services for students with disabilities lead me to make the following recommendations for future evaluators:

1. Approach the evaluation enterprise with a clear purpose in mind, determining whether the primary intent is to ensure accountability or program improvement.
2. Advocate for development of multiple approaches at the state and national levels that support local level decision making without compromising state level data integrity.
3. Use incentives and sanctions cautiously.
4. Interpret data based on evaluations of conceptual models that show the expected linkages among the inputs, processes and outcomes of each educational service and experience that affect students with disabilities.

5. Define effectiveness indicators and outcomes for students with disabilities within the context of outcomes for all students, ensuring that the unique needs of students with disabilities for access, accommodation, adaptation and compensation are addressed.

We can benefit from the developments and experiences of the past. Doing so could mean that another retrospective such as this in the year 2009 might describe a state-of-affairs in which adequate information on the progress of students with disabilities is being documented and used within a comprehensive evaluation framework for all of education.

REFERENCES

Accreditation Council on Services for People with Disabilities. (1993). *Outcome based performance measures.* Landover, MD: Author.

Bickel, W. E., & Bickel, D. D. (1986). Effective schools, classrooms, and instruction: Implications for special education. *Exceptional Children, 52*(6), 489-500.

Borich, G. D. (1977). Program evaluation: New concept, new methods. *Focus on Exceptional Children, 9*(3), 1-14.

Borich, G. D., & Nance, D. D. (1987). Evaluating special education programs: Shifting the professional mandate from process to outcome. *Remedial and Special Education, 8*(3), 7-16.

Brinkerhoff, R. O., Brethower, D. M., Hluchyj, T., & Nowakowski, J. R. (1983). *Program evaluation: A practitioner's guide for trainers and educators–design manual.* Boston, MA: Kluwer-Nijhoff Publishing.

California Office of Special Education. (1982). *Guide to special education program evaluation.* Sacramento, CA: California State Department of Education.

Campeau, P. (1993). *Project PASS (Performance assessment for self-sufficiency).* Palo Alto, CA: American Institutes for Research.

Center for Policy Options in Special Education. (1992). *Policy issues and elements: Outcomes-based accountability,* Rockville, MD: WESTAT.

Chen, H. (1990). Issues in constructing program theory. *New directions for program evaluation: Advances in program theory (No. 47).* San Francisco, CA: Jossey-Bass, Publishers.

COSMOS. (1994). *The National Agenda for achieving better results for children and youth with disabilities.* Washington, DC: Author.

DeStefano, L. (1990). Evaluating effectiveness: Federal expectations and local capabilities. *Studies in Educational Evaluation, 16,* 257-269.

DeStefano, L., & Wagner, M. (1990). *Outcome assessment in special education: Lessons learned.* Champaign, IL: Transition Institute at Illinois.

Frey, W. D. (1991). *Outcome indicators for special education: A model for studying the expected outcomes of education for students with disabilities.* East Lansing, MI: Center for Quality Special Education.

Fullan, M. (1991). *The new meaning of educational change* (2nd ed.). New York: Teachers College Press, Columbia University.

Gable, R. K. (1982). A model for evaluating special education programs: An application to determining the management and instructional benefits of microcomputers. *Journal of Special Education Technology, 5*(2), 35-43.

Gartner, A., & Lipsky, D. K. (1989). *The yoke of special education: How to break it.* New York: National Center on Education and the Economy.

George, M. P., George, N. L., & Grosenick, J.K. (1990). Features of program evaluation in special education. *Remedial and Special Education, 11*(5), 23-30.

Gonzales, P. (1992). *State procedures for the evaluation of special education program effectiveness.* Washington, DC: Project FORUM, National Association of State Directors of Special Education.

Halvorsen, A. T., & Sailor, W. (1989). *Integration of students with severe and profound disabilities: A review of research.* California Research Institute on the Integration of Students with Severe Disabilities.

Hasazi, S. B., Hock, M., & Cravedi-Cheng, L. (1993). *Vermont's post school indicators project: Dissemination materials.* Burlington, VT: Vermont's Transition Systems Change Project.

Horvath, L. J. (1985). A quantitative program evaluation approach to evaluating quality special education programs. In *Quantitative vs. qualitative approaches to quality special education program evaluation* (pp. 3-20). Bloomington, IN: Council of Administrators of Special Education.

Horvath, L. J. (1992). *Educating policy makers on the importance of a comprehensive evaluation approach.* Presentation at the American Evaluation Association Annual Meeting, Seattle, WA, November 5, 1992.

Illinois State Board of Education. (1982). *Handbook for evaluation of special education effectiveness.* Springfield, IL: Author.

Jefferson County Public Schools. (1988). *Best practice standards for the teacher of the exceptional child.* Louisville, KY: Author.

Kleinert, H., Smith, P., & Hudson, M. (1990). *Quality program indicators manual for students with moderate and severe handicaps.* Lexington, KY: University of Kentucky, Interdisciplinary Human Development Institute: Kentucky System Change Project for Students with Severe Handicaps.

Lachat, M. A., Williams, M., & Brody, S. (1986). *Profiling effectiveness in special education: A program improvement system based on indicators of effectiveness.* Hampton, NH: Center for Resource Management.

Lewis, A. (1991). Churning up the waters in special education. *Phi Delta Kappan, 73*(2) 100-101.

Lieberman, L. M., & McNeil, D. (1982). Evaluating special education programs. *Journal of Learning Disabilities, 15*(2), 121-122.

Little, D. L. (1993) *Outcome-based education and students with learning disabilities.* Chapel Hill, NC: University of North Carolina.

Maher, C. A., & Bennett, R. E. (1983). A systems framework for special education program evaluation. *Diagnostique, 8*(4), 203-212.

Maher, C. A., & Bennett, R. E. (1984) *Planning and evaluating special education services.* Englewood Cliffs, NJ: Prentice-Hall, Inc.

Massachusetts Division of Special Education. (1981). *Special education program evaluation: A management tool.* Quincy, MA: Massachusetts Department of Education.

McLaughlin, J. A. (1988). *Special education program evaluation: An overview.* Bloomington, IN: Council of Administrators of Special Education (CASE) Research Committee.

Missouri Section of Special Education. (1985). *Special education evaluation model for Missouri.* Columbia, MO: Missouri Department of Elementary and Secondary Education.

Nance, D., & Borich, G. (1986). *Manual for the special education evaluation system: Compliance, coordination, and change measures.* Austin, TX: The Special Education Evaluation Institute.

NASBE. (1992). *Winners all: A call for inclusive schools.* Alexandria, VA: National Association of State Boards of Education.

National Council on Disability. (1989). *The education of students with disabilities: Where do we stand?–A report to the president of the congress of the United States.* Washington, DC: National Council on Disability.

National RRC Panel on Indicators of Effectiveness in Special Education. (1986). *Effectiveness indicators for special education: A reference tool.* Lexington, KY: University of Kentucky, Mid-South Regional Resource Center.

North Carolina Division for Exceptional Children. (1983). *Special education program quality evaluation.* Raleigh, NC: North Carolina Department of Public Instruction.

Olsen, K. (1979). *Evaluating effectiveness of special education programs.* Lexington, KY: University of Kentucky, Mid-South Regional Resource Center.

Olsen, K. (1984). *State program evaluation in special education: Issues, practices and some reflections.* Lexington, KY: University of Kentucky, Mid-South Regional Resource Center.

Olsen, K. (1986). *State program evaluation efforts: Needs and approaches.* Lexington, KY: University of Kentucky, Mid-South Regional Resource Center.

Olsen, K. (1994). *What we know about using data to lead change.* Presentation at the National Agenda Conference, Washington, DC, July 11, 1994.

Olsen, K. R., & Massanari, C. (1991). *Special education program evaluation: What should states consider?* Lexington, KY: University of Kentucky, Mid-South Regional Resource Center.

Olsen, K. R., & Turley, C. R. (1988). *Description of effective special education programs in West Virginia: A reference tool for the special education effectiveness review (SEER) system.* Lexington, KY: University of Kentucky, Mid-South Regional Resource Center.

Porter, A. (1993). Defining and measuring opportunity to learn in *The debate on opportunity-to-learn standards: Supporting Works*. Papers commissioned by the National Governor's Association, Washington, DC.

Rhode Island Department of Education. (1984). *A self-study guide for the evaluation of special education programs*. Providence, RI: Author.

Robert Wood Johnson Foundation. (1988). *Serving handicapped children: A special report*. Princeton, NJ: Author.

Rogers, E. (1983). *Diffusion of innovations* (3rd ed.). New York: The Free Press (Division of Macmillan Publishing Co. Inc.).

Stainback, S., & Stainback, W. (1984). A rational for the merger of special and regular education. *Exceptional Children, 51*(2), 102-111.

Utah Consortium of Local Directors of Special Education. (1988). *Utah special education evaluation system (Utah SEES)*. Utah: Author.

Vogelsberg, R. T. (1994). Educational reform, inclusion, and special education: Are we focused on student outcomes? *Quality Outcomes-Driven Education, 3*(4), 24-31.

Wagner, M. (1990). *Young people with disabilities: How are they doing?—A comprehensive report from Wave I of the National Longitudinal Transition Study of Special Education Students*. Menlo Park, CA: SRI International.

Ysseldyke, J., Thurlow, M., Bruininks, R., Gilman, C., Deno, S., McGrew, K., & Shriner, J. (1992). *An evolving model of educational outcomes for children and youth with disabilities* (Working Paper 2). Minneapolis, MN: University of Minnesota, National Center on Educational Outcomes.

Ysseldyke, J., Thurlow, M., McGrew, K., & Vanderwood, M. (1994). *Making decisions about the inclusion of students with disabilities in large-scale assessments: A report on a working conference to develop guidelines on inclusion and accommodations* (Synthesis Report 13). Minneapolis, MN: University of Minnesota, National Center on Educational Outcomes.

Ysseldyke, J., Thurlow, M., & Shriner, J. G. (1992). Outcomes are for special educators too. *Teaching Exceptional Children, 25*(1), 36-50.

Zirkel, P. A. (1990, August 31). 'Backlash' threatens special education. *Education Week*.

What Results Should Be Measured
to Decide Whether Instruction
Is Working for Students with Disabilities?

James E. Ysseldyke
Martha L. Thurlow

National Center on Educational Outcomes
University of Minnesota

SUMMARY. Current educational reform activities and cries for accountability are generating considerable discussion and debate about what the important results of education should be. The controversy that often surrounds this discussion spills over to discussions about what we should measure. In this article, we describe the process that the National Center on Educational Outcomes used to generate outcomes, and indicators of those outcomes, that could be viewed as applying to *all* students. The descriptions of the process are designed to provide special services personnel with a perspective on how they might be leaders in developing school goals and standards for students.

The development of this article was supported in part by a Cooperative Agreement (H159C00004) between the University of Minnesota and the U.S. Department of Education, Office of Special Education Programs. Points of view or opinions expressed in the article are not necessarily those of the department or offices within it.

Address correspondence to: James E. Ysseldyke, 350 Elliott Hall, 75 East River Road, University of Minnesota, Minneapolis, MN 55455.

[Haworth co-indexing entry note]: "What Results Should Be Measured to Decide Whether Instruction Is Working for Students with Disabilities?" Ysseldyke, James E., and Martha L. Thurlow. Co-published simultaneously in *Special Services in the Schools* (The Haworth Press, Inc.) Vol. 9, No. 2, 1994, pp. 39-49; and: *Educational Outcomes for Students with Disabilities* (ed: James E. Ysseldyke, and Martha L. Thurlow) The Haworth Press, Inc., 1994, pp. 39-49. Multiple copies of this article/chapter may be purchased from The Haworth Document Delivery Center [1-800-3-HAWORTH; 9:00 a.m. - 5:00 p.m. (EST)].

39

School personnel are under considerable pressure to demonstrate that their instructional efforts are producing desired results. That push comes from several directions, and is a result of multiple forces, singly and in interaction.

There is a tendency to attribute decline in the U.S. standard of living and economic competitiveness to a decline in the quality of schools (Goodlad, 1992). Since publication of *A Nation At Risk* in the early '80s (National Commission on Excellence in Education, 1983), there have been a series of critiques of U.S. schools and a series of calls for reform, restructuring and reorganizing to promote excellence. Schools are busy restructuring and reforming. Primarily they do this so students will benefit from education more than they are now, and so that schools will achieve better results.

The cry for higher standards, greater degrees of excellence, and better results is accompanied by much debate about the kinds of results schools are attempting to or expected to achieve. How do we know whether schools get better? How are we to know whether students achieve as much as they possibly can, or whether they achieve what we want them to achieve? How do taxpayers know whether they are getting their money's worth from public schools? How do school board members know whether their schools are delivering what is expected, which schools are performing well, which teachers are doing a good job? How do teachers know whether their students achieve the results they expect?

The quick response to the questions posed is "test students." Further deliberation of the questions leads to responses like "demonstrate accountability," "prepare report cards on schools," "measure pupil performance," "set high standards and measure achievement of them," and "chart pupil progress toward accomplishment of objectives." But, what objectives, what standards, what outcomes? What results should schools and teachers try to achieve? The questions go to the very heart of what schools are about. The questions call for careful definition, for delineation of the skills, knowledge, attitudes, values and behaviors that schools try to inculcate in pupils. In this article, we consider development of a conceptual methodology for assessment of results or outcomes for students with disabilities.

There clearly is much debate about what to account for in the development of indices of accountability. And, in fact, one obtains different answers to the "What should we measure?" question as a function of the group one asks. Examples of alternative responses to this question are listed in Table 1. We list outcomes specified as part of Goals 2000, work-identified outcomes, general education identified outcomes, and special education identified outcomes. In September 1993, we convened a group of State Directors of Special Education and State Assessment Directors. A question was posed to the group: "What data would you need to document the extent to which education is working for students with disabilities?" Those in attendance at the meeting generated the list of outcomes variables shown in Table 2. They also identified input data and indices of the educational process they said they would need to make decisions. Note the range of kinds of information desired. Participants did not rank order the information in terms of priority.

Much of the debate about results or outcomes is focused on nonacademic outcomes (see article by Shriner in this volume). Much of that debate is as much about who ought to decide and measure as it is about what ought to be taught and measured. The debate about nonacademic outcomes (the teaching of attitudes, values and beliefs) is neither new nor unanticipated.

Historically, many of the discussions about the outcomes of schooling have been discipline-specific. Educators talk about cognitive, affective, social, and vocational outcomes. Some psychologists talk about "megaskills" like confidence, motivation, effort, responsibility, initiative, caring, perseverance and common sense (Rich, 1988). Other psychologists talk about outcomes like physical competence, adaptive intelligence, and social competence. Sociologists talk about social skills, life maintenance skills, basic literacy, and attitudes. Mental health practitioners talk about outcomes like closeness, trusting, dealing with frustration, handling separation and independence, working for delayed gratification, and cognitive processing, among others (Strayhorn, 1988).

The National Center on Educational Outcomes (NCEO) has been working over the past three years with state and federal education agencies to facilitate and enrich the development and use of indicators of educational outcomes for students with disabilities. The use of outcomes and indicators should improve educational results for

TABLE 1. Outcomes Identified by Different Groups

National Education Goals (Goals 2000)	Work-Identified Outcomes

• School Readiness
• Graduation
• Achievement
• Teacher Preparation
• Science and Math Excellence
• Literacy (Lifelong Learning)
• Safe, Disciplined, Drug-Free Schools
• Parent Involvement
	What Work Requires of Schools (1991)[a]
	• Competencies: Can productively use
	  * Resources
	  * Interpersonal Skills
	  * Information
	  * Systems
	  * Technology
	• Foundations for Competencies
	  * Basic Skills
	  * Thinking Skills
	  * Personal Qualities

General Education-Identified Outcomes	**Special Education-Identified Outcomes**
Council of Chief State School Officers (1990)[b] • Attendance • Achievement • Attainment • Affective Status • Post-School Status **National Forum on Education Statistics (1990)[c]** • Achievement • Participation • Dropout Rate • Attitudes • Aspirations **Special Study Panel on Educational Indicators (1991)[d]** • Achievement • Attainment • Postsecondary Experiences • Beyond School Experiences	**Mid-South Regional Resource Center (1986)[e]** • Student Performance • Competencies • Behaviors and Attitudes • Satisfaction • Post-School Status **SRI National Longitudinal Transition Study (1989)[f]** • Education • Employment • Independent Living • Postsecondary and Adult Services • Postsecondary Status **National Council on Disability (1990)[g]** • Academic Achievement • Work Readiness • Quality of Life (internal and external)

[a] *State Education Indicators 1990* by the Council of Chief State School Officers, Washington, DC (1990).

[b] *A Guide to Improving the National Education Data Systems* by the National Forum on Education Statistics, National Center for Education Statistics, Washington, DC (1990).

[c] *Education Counts: An Indicator System to Monitor the Nation's Educational Health* by the Special Study Panel on Education Indicators, National Center for Education Statistics, Washington, DC (1991).

[d] *Effectiveness Indicators for Special Education a Reference Tool* by the Mid-South Regional Resource Center, Lexington, KY (1986).

[e] *The Education of Students with Disabilities: Where Do We Stand?* by the National Council on Disability, Washington, DC (1989).

[g] *What Work Requires of Schools: A SCANS Report for America 2000* by the Secretary's Commission on Achieving Necessary Skills, U.S. Department of Labor, Washington, DC (1991).

TABLE 2. Data Educators Need to Make Judgements About Whether Education Is Working for Students

Input Data

Resources (e.g., money spent per pupil, staffing ratio, instructional time)

Student Characteristics (e.g., percentage of first graders with kindergarten experience, student mobility, number of LEP students, Chapter 1 students, Special Education students, number on free/reduced price meal)

Process Data

Opportunity to Learn

Inclusion of Students with Disabilities in General Education

Teacher Expectations for Individual Pupil Performance

Extent to Which IEPs Translate into Instruction

Outcomes Data

Academic and Functional Skills

Valued Social and Emotional Outcomes

Generalization of School Learning to Everyday Life

Student and Parent Satisfaction

Independent Living

Community Participation

Extent to Which the "Product" of Schools Meets the Needs of the Labor Market all students. One of the major activities of the NCEO has been the development of a comprehensive conceptual model of educational outcomes and indicators. The Center has been engaged in a variety of activities designed to produce the conceptual model, a comprehensive set of outcomes, and indicators. Our objective has been to develop consensus on those outcomes that ought to be assessed. We have gone through a number of steps in reaching agreement on a model of outcomes and indicators.

In our work at NCEO we initially proposed to develop separate models from different disciplinary perspectives and then to develop outcomes, indicators, and measures specific to each model. We thought we would do so as a function of severity of disability and the age level of the student. Currently our approach differs significantly from our original intent.

DEFINITIONAL CONSIDERATIONS

Other articles in this special volume speak to the importance of clear definitions of terms in discussions about outcomes. We found that this was critical. NCEO staff began the model development process by developing definitions of the terms "outcomes" and "indicators." First, we reviewed definitions proposed in the professional literature by researchers and policymakers. We then reached agreement among our own staff on the definition of outcomes (the results of interactions among individuals and schooling experiences). We defined what we meant by interactions, schooling experiences, individuals, and results. An indicator was defined as "a symbolic representation of one or more educational outcomes for infants, children and youth that enables comparisons to be made." We then generated a set of assumptions to guide the model development efforts. These were:

1. Indicators of outcomes in special education should be related conceptually and statistically to those that are useful generally in education.
2. Educational outcomes indicators must provide data needed to make policy decisions primarily at school, state, and national levels, but possess implications for evaluating educational programs at other levels.

3. Outcomes indicators are most useful when they are functionally related to educational inputs, contextual characteristics, and to processes.

In February 1990, we met with six state directors of special education. We provided them with a preliminary draft of Working Paper 1, which included definitions, assumptions, and a new model. The directors responded to our article. Following that meeting, NCEO staff presented the definitions, assumptions, and proposed model as part of an article at a major conference sponsored by the Connecticut Department of Education and designed to look at the future of education for students with disabilities. Formal feedback was received on the model and indicators from those in attendance at the conference.

NCEO personnel developed a working paper delineating definitions of terms, assumptions, and a proposed model of outcomes (Ysseldyke, Thurlow, Bruininks, Deno, McGrew, & Shriner, 1991) and sent this to selected representatives of professional associations and to all state directors of special education. The paper was reviewed formally at meetings in Montana, Michigan, and Nebraska. Responses to the working paper were gathered for about a six month period and are synthesized in a document entitled "Synthesis of Responses to Working Paper 1" (Gilman, Thurlow, & Ysseldyke, 1992). The models of educational outcomes proposed in the first Working Paper are illustrated in Figure 1.

Between the time of our initial work and the development of Working Paper 2, we developed the concept of "enabling outcomes." These were defined as "the results of interactions between individuals and life experiences that provide individuals with the opportunity to reach educational outcomes."

THE MODEL DEVELOPMENT PROCESS

In December 1991, NCEO convened a meeting of individuals who had previously engaged in considerable activity relevant to the development of outcomes and indicators in representative states. At that meeting we used a multi-attribute consensus-building process (Vanderwood & Erickson, this volume) to generate outcomes and

FIGURE 1. Proposed Models of Educational Outcomes (Ysseldyke et al., 1991)

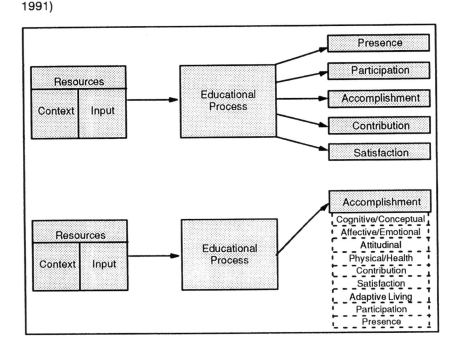

indicators, engage in editing of outcomes and indicators, and reach agreement upon outcomes and indicators in each of the domains in the then-current model. In April 1992, we met with a group of parents, school personnel, and representatives of advocacy groups. We engaged in a multi-attribute consensus building process in an effort to have those individuals generate outcomes, indicators, and indicate their importance.

In April 1992, personnel from NCEO presented a paper at the annual Leadership Conference held by the Office of Special Education Programs. The definitions of the terms "outcomes" and "indicators" were presented, assumptions were presented, unresolved issues were described, and the model was presented. Reaction was received from state directors of special education and others in attendance at that meeting.

In May 1992, a meeting was held in Minneapolis with six state directors of special education. Once again a multi-attribute consensus building process was used to arrive at agreement on outcomes and indicators for each of the domains in the model at grade 12.

In September 1992, members of the NCEO staff published a paper in *Exceptional Children* (Ysseldyke, Thurlow, & Shriner, 1992) based on the model. The model at that time is shown in Figure 2. Also in September 1992 we convened a meeting in Washington, DC that was attended by representatives of more than 20 agencies or groups. At that meeting we engaged once again in a multi-attribute consensus building process designed to reach agreement on indicators of educational outcomes for school completion. The model evolved to the one illustrated in Figure 3. The specific set of outcomes and indicators generated were then reviewed by those in attendance and compiled into a document entitled "Educational Outcomes and Indicators for Students Completing School." The document was reviewed by several selected Directors of Special Education. Modifications were made and the document was published in February 1993 (Ysseldyke, Thurlow & Gilman, 1993).

A final step in the development of a conceptual model was the preparation of a self study guide for states and districts to use in development of their own model of outcomes and indicators (see paper by Thurlow, Ysseldyke, Vanderwood & Spade, this volume). It was thought that it would not be a good idea simply to suggest to state education agency personnel that they use the model we derived. Rather, it was thought that we should prepare a document taking educators through a set of steps in model development.

CONCLUSION

This article was developed both to document the process NCEO used in the development of its model of educational outcomes, and to provide special services personnel with a perspective on how they might be leaders in the outcomes development process. This is a process that can by used by school staff to develop school goals, standards, or to provide feedback to model developers.

FIGURE 2. Revised Model of Educational Outcomes (Ysseldyke et al., 1992)

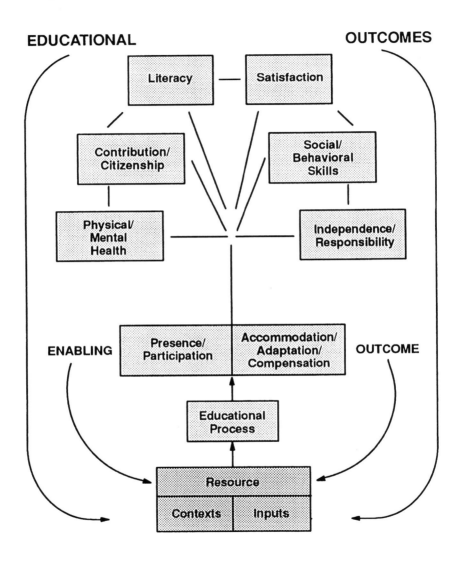

FIGURE 3. School Completion Model (Ysseldyke et al., 1993)

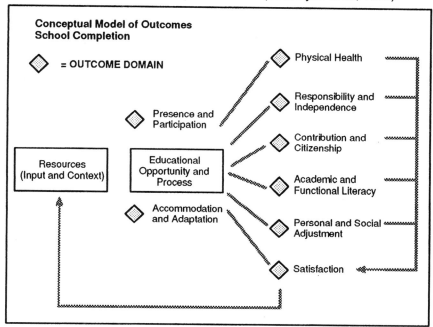

REFERENCES

Gilman, C., Thurlow, M.L., & Ysseldyke, J.E. (1992). *Synthesis of working paper 1.* Minneapolis, MN: National Center on Educational Outcomes.

Goodlad, J. (1992). On taking school reform seriously. *Phi Delta Kappan, 74,* 232-238.

National Commission on Excellence in Education. (1983). *A nation at risk: The imperative for educational reform.* Washington, D.C.: U.S. Government Printing office.

Rich, D. (1988). *MegaSkills: How families can help children succeed in school and beyond.* Boston: Houghton-Mifflin Co.

Strayhorn, J. (1988). *The competent child.* New York: Guilford Press.

Ysseldyke, J.E., Thurlow, M.L., Bruininks, R.H., Deno, S.L., McGrew, K., & Shriner, J. (1991). *A conceptual model of educational outcomes and indicators for students with disabilities. Working Paper #1.* Minneapolis, MN: National Center on Educational Outcomes.

Ysseldyke, J.E., Thurlow, M.L., & Gilman, C. (1993). *Educational outcomes and indicators for students completing school.* Minneapolis, MN: National Center on Educational Outcomes.

Ysseldyke, J.E., Thurlow, M.L., & Shriner, J. (1992). Outcomes are for special educators too. *Teaching Exceptional Children, 25,* 36-50.

National Outcome Data Collection Programs: How They Can Be Used at the Local Level

Kevin S. McGrew

St. Cloud State University

SUMMARY. The current wave of education reform has focused significant attention at the state and national level on measurement-driven accountability and evaluation. This article introduces special services personnel to the major national data collection agencies and select data collection programs that provide outcome indicators that monitor the health of our education system. The goal is to encourage special services personnel to become informed consumers and participants in education reform dialogues. In addition, it is suggested that local evaluation activities can be significantly improved by borrowing portions of national data collection survey instruments. Information is presented on how to secure the necessary information to make use of national data collection information at the local education level.

The development of this article was supported in part by a Cooperative Agreement (H159C00004) between the University of Minnesota and the U.S. Department of Education, Office of Special Education Programs. Points of view or opinions expressed in the article are not necessarily those of the department or offices within it.

Address correspondence to: Kevin S. McGrew, St. Cloud State University, Department of Applied Psychology, 720 4th Avenue South, St. Cloud, MN 56301.

[Haworth co-indexing entry note]: "National Outcome Data Collection Programs: How They Can Be Used at the Local Level." McGrew, Kevin S. Co-published simultaneously in *Special Services in the Schools* (The Haworth Press, Inc.) Vol. 9, No. 2, 1994, pp. 51-62; and: *Educational Outcomes for Students with Disabilities* (ed: James E. Ysseldyke, and Martha L. Thurlow) The Haworth Press, Inc., 1994, pp. 51-62. Multiple copies of this article/chapter may be purchased from The Haworth Document Delivery Center [1-800-3-HAWORTH; 9:00 a.m. - 5:00 p.m. (EST)].

51

Calls for reform in American education during the past decade have resulted in raised expectations, attempts to develop "world class" standards, and increased interest in the measurement of school outcomes. The current wave of education reform has focused significant attention on measurement-driven accountability and evaluation. "School reform has riveted national attention on the numbers" (Hanford & White, 1991).

At state and national levels, attention has focused on the use of large-scale assessment programs (e.g., National Assessment of Educational Progress; state minimum competency testing programs) to measure the results or outcomes of education and reform activities (McGrew, Spiegel, Thurlow, Ysseldyke, Bruininks, & Shriner, 1992). Results from these assessment programs often appear in local and national newspapers in the form of eye-catching headlines such as: "Eighth grade students in state X rank 20th in the nation in mathematics," "Only X percent of all high school graduates can complete a job application form," or "X percent of junior high students experience violence or harassment during school."

Educators and parents are often intrigued by these reports and ask: "I wonder if the same thing is happening with the children in our school or community?" Similar questions often are asked more formally at the local level as the result of state or locally required public evaluation and reporting activities. However, it is only when a media report highlights a startling education statistic, particularly when focused on the specific state or local education agency (LEA) where an educator lives, that LEA staff usually pay attention to national data collection activities. Unfortunately, this attention is frequently short lived.

LEA personnel need to become intelligent consumers of the large mass of information provided by recurring national education data collection programs in order to: (a) become informed participants in local, state, and national dialogues on education reform, (b) become cognizant of national level events that can influence the development and education of children and youth, and (c) improve the level of sophistication, including possible LEA comparisons to national statistics, of local evaluation activities. The purpose of this article is to introduce special services personnel to the existence and potential use of information available from select national data collection programs.

WHO GATHERS THE NATIONAL DATA?

Most Americans, whether they are in education or not, have an awareness of the most visible national data collection program–the "census." Every 10 years, the U. S. Bureau of the Census conducts a comprehensive survey of the U. S. population. In addition, the Bureau of the Census conducts smaller annual supplemental surveys of representative samples of the U. S. population. These recurring surveys produce information on demographic and other critical characteristics (e.g., employment and income statistics) of the U. S. population.

Not all educators are aware that there is a similar federal agency that collects and reports routine data on the status of education in the U. S. The National Center for Education Statistics (NCES) is the Department of Education's analog to the Bureau of the Census. NCES "collects statistics on the condition of education in the United States, analyzes and reports the meaning and significance of these statistics, and assists states and local education agencies in improving their statistical systems" (NCES, 1991). NCES fulfills this function by sponsoring and directing a variety of cross-sectional and longitudinal data collection programs at the elementary, secondary, and postsecondary education levels. Although each data collection program produces many reports, the NCES annually publishes three major publications that are widely circulated and that should be reviewed by special services and other LEA personnel. These are *The Condition of Education,* the *Digest of Education Statistics,* and *Projections of Education Statistics.*

The National Center on Educational Outcomes (NCEO) for students with disabilities has identified over two dozen national data collection programs that include indicators of important educational outcomes for all students (Ysseldyke, Thurlow, Bruininks, Gilman, Deno, McGrew, & Shriner, 1992). Five of the most prominent Department of Education sponsored data collection programs identified by the NCEO are listed and described in Table 1. Included in the descriptions are a brief list of the general variable domains assessed by each data collection program. A more detailed analysis of the individual items or questions included in each data collection program, organized according to the NCEO School Completion model of outcomes and indicators (see Ysseldyke and Thurlow in this volume) is available (McGrew, Spiegel, Thurlow, & Kim, 1994).

Although indicators of important educational outcomes (Ysseldyke et al., 1992) are systematically gathered as part of national data collection programs sponsored by other federal departments (viz., Departments of Commerce, Labor, and Justice), the Department of Health and Human Services, primarily through the National Center for Health Statistics (NCHS), sponsors the next largest number of data collection programs that include indicators of important outcomes related to the NCEO conceptual model (McGrew et al., 1992). A listing and brief description of three select Department of Health and Human Services data programs is presented in Table 2.

WHAT CAN I LEARN FROM NATIONAL DATA COLLECTION PROGRAMS?

At a time of increased decentralization of educational decision making through site-based management, there is the opposite trend toward the centralization of the measurement and evaluation of education outcomes at both the national and state levels. The analysis of educational indicators from national education data sets is increasing. The intent of these analyses is to produce policy-relevant reports that can guide program improvement and accountability activities, help with the formulation of educational policy, and inform the public about how well the nation's schools are serving children and youth.

Although the development and reporting of an overall "educational health index" similar to the Dow Jones Index, the Consumer Price Index, or the Gross National Product is not likely, educational outcome indicator data are rapidly becoming the language of current education reform discussions. Just as these other national indexes and indicators often generate a flurry of discussion and resulting action, critical policy makers are using the increasing amount of national education indicator information to make decisions that can have significant and longstanding impact on the

TABLE 1. Descriptions of Select National Data Collection Programs Sponsored by the Department of Education

---

National Adult Literacy Survey (NALS)
A nationally representative cross-sectional study to collect information on types and levels of literacy skills of adults. This data collection program assesses (a) prose, document, and quantitative literacy, (b) language, employment, and education background and experiences, (c) social and political participation, and (d) literacy activities.

National Assessment of Educational Progress (NAEP)
A nationally representative cross-sectional study to monitor the knowledge, skills, understanding, and attitudes of children and youth. This data collection program assesses different curriculum areas (e.g., reading, writing, mathematics) in grades 4, 8, and 12. A voluntary state program (Trial State Assessment Program) started in1990. In addition to student performance, this data collection program assesses (a) school characteristics and policy infomation, (b) teacher characteristics, (c) classroom curriculum and teaching methods, and (d) subject-specific student background and attitude information.

National Education Longitudinal Study (NELS)
A nationally representative longitudinal study to assess the baseline school and non-school experiences of 8th grade students in 1988 and to relate these to academic achievement and to later achievement in school and life, with assessments every two years to 1996.

National Household Education Survey (NHES)
A nationally representative cross-sectional study of households to examine early and adult education issues. The 1991 base year survey collected information on the care, and education of 3 to 8 year old children, and the participation of adults in education activities. Other targeted information includes (a) home environment, (b) health and disability characteristics of young children, (c) parent and adult education and employment, and (d) previous and current educational background and participation of adults.

National Longitudinal Transition Study of Special Education Students (NLTS)
A nationally representative longitudinal study of *special education students* who were in grades 7-12 during the 1987 base year sample. By collecting a wide array of information from parents/guardians, school records, and school administrators, this data collection program provides descriptive information regarding the transition of youth with disabilities from secondary school to early adulthood, and seeks to identify factors that contribute to effective transition of youth with disabilities. The first follow-up was completed in 1990.

TABLE 2. Descriptions of Select National Data Collection Programs Sponsored by the Department of Health and Human Services

---

Monitoring the Future (MTF)
A nationally representative cross-sectional study of 8th, 10th, and 12th grade students to annually assess the preference, values, and changing life-styles of students. This data collection program assesses (a) drug behaviors, attitudes, and related factors, (b) high school educational and employment experiences, role behaviors, and satisfactions, and (c) social values, attitudes, and behaviors.

National Adolescent Student Health Survey (NASHS)
A nationally representative cross-sectional study of 8th and 10th grade students to assess attitudes toward (a) nutrition and consumer health, (b) AIDS and sexually transmitted disease, (c) tobacco, drug, and alcohol use, (d) suicide and violence, and (e) injury prevention.

Youth Risk Behavior Survey (YRBS)
A nationally representative cross-sectional study of students in grades 9-12 that is part of the Youth Risk Behavior Surveillance System (YRBSS). This study assesses every two years the prevalence of priority health-risk behaviors, including (a) intentional and unintentional injurious behavior, (b) tobacco, alcohol, and other drug use, (c) sexual behaviors, (d) dietary behaviors, and (e) physical activity.

---

education of children. Given that the results of these national data collection programs are disseminated in free or low cost reports, LEA staff can become familiar with the same information being provided to critical decision makers (e.g., legislators, policymakers) by simply requesting this information.

Although national activities often appear to have little direct relevance to the day-to-day activities of LEA personnel, the results of these activities, most often in the form of legislation, policy decisions, and resource allocation, can have a significant indirect impact on each local school. According to the ecological systems perspective (Bronfenbrenner, 1979), to fully appreciate the how and why of the development of children and youth, one needs to be aware of all the proximal and direct (e.g., family relationships, home environment), distal and indirect (e.g., changes in one's culture, changes in federal education policy that impacts resource allocation), and intermediate (e.g., community characteristics and resources, informal social support networks, changes at the local school) influences that can affect the development of children and youth. By keeping abreast of nationally based reports, many that are written in understandable formats for public consumption, LEA personnel can develop a better appreciation of the "big picture" of U. S. education. Equipped with this knowledge, an informed consumer can participate in important dialogues that occur at the local, state, and national levels regarding education. National indicator data are the primary language of the current education reform dialogues. LEA personnel need to develop their "National Indicator Data as a Second Language" (NIDSL) competencies in order to understand and participate in these important activities. All that is required is a short letter or phone call to get on the appropriate federal dissemination mailing lists.

HOW CAN WE GATHER COMPARABLE DATA AT THE LOCAL LEVEL?

A direct advantage of increased NIDSL competency is the possibility of using components of national data collection instruments for local evaluation activities. Although access to the formal tests of achievement included in many national data collection programs is not possible for test security reasons, most of the non-test data gathering components (e.g., student, teacher, parent completed questionnaires or surveys) are in the public domain. One simply needs to request or order the appropriate manual or report (often at a very minimal cost) that includes copies of the actual survey instruments.

In local evaluation activities, LEA staff often develop their own survey instruments. Unless the local school system employs professionals with program evaluation expertise, many times the final instruments vary widely in technical adequacy. Also, the development of sound survey questions can be very time consuming and expensive. By using national data collection program survey items, LEA staff can dramatically increase the technical adequacy of their evaluation activities at a minimal cost. Many of these national survey items have direct relevance to local evaluation activities. Select items from the National Education Longitudinal Study (NELS) and the Youth Risk Behavior Survey (YRBS) are presented for illustrative purposes in Table 3.

TABLE 3. Select Sample Items from Two National Data Collection Programs

---

National Education Longitudinal Survey (NELS)

How do you feel about each of the following statements?
(responses on a 4-point rating scale)

  a. I feel good about myself
  b. I don't have enough control over the direction my life is taking
  c. In my life, good luck is more important than hard work for success
  d. I feel I am a person of worth, the equal of other people
  e. I am able to do things as well as most other people
  f. Every time I try to get ahead, something or somebody stops me
  g. My plans hardly ever work out, so planning only makes me unhappy
  h. On the whole, I am satisfied with myself
  i. I feel useless at times
  j. At times, I think I am no good at all
  k. When I make plans, I am almost certain I can make them work
  l. I feel I do not have much to be proud of
  m. Chance and luck are very important for what happens in my life

Youth Risk Behavior Survey (YRBS)

During the past 30 days, how many times did you ride in a car or other vehicle driven by someone who had been drinking?

  a. 0 times
  b. 1 time
  c. 2 or 3 times
  d. 4 or 5 times
  e. 6 or more times

During the past 30 days, how many days did you *not* go to school because you felt you would be unsafe at school or on your way to or from school?

  a. 0 days
  b. 1 day
  c. 2 or 3 days
  d. 4 or 5 days
  e. 6 or more days

The samples presented in Table 3 are items completed by students. Accommodations or adaptations may be necessary for students who have the cognitive capabilities to understand self-report survey questions, but who have a disability that precludes independent completion (e.g., severe reading disability). Many national data collection programs also contain surveys that are completed by third-party informants (viz., teachers and parents). Parent and teacher completed surveys may be particularly useful for assessing those students with disabilities who are unable to complete the self-report measures.

There is a rich source of survey items potentially available for local use. For example, across 13 national data collection programs that provide information at the school completion level, the NCEO found that 70 of 77 (91%) indicators included in the NCEO school completion outcomes and indicators model could be found across the major outcome domains (e.g., presence and participation, accommodation and adaptation, physical health, responsibility and independence, contribution and citizenship, academic and functional literacy, personal and social adjustment, and satisfaction) (McGrew et al., 1994). For LEA personnel interested in the assessment of outcomes at the completion of school, the McGrew et al. (1994) document contains detailed tables that indicate which data collection programs contain specific NCEO school completion indicators. Future reports at other developmental levels are forthcoming from the NCEO.

Items in national data collection instruments are developed through a systematic process by measurement professionals. The items have typically undergone significant field-testing and debugging. Thus, by "borrowing" those national survey items or components that are relevant to a local evaluation need, LEA staff can save significant time and can feel more comfortable in the technical adequacy of the items used.

More importantly, by using the same survey items and consulting the final national reports, LEA staff may be able to compare how their local data compare to national results. For example, on a NELS item that asked students whether the possession of weapons is a problem in their school, 11.1% and 10.1% of a nationally representative sample of 10th grade students in 1990 reported this to be a "serious" or "moderate" problem, respectively (Ingels, Scott, Lindmark, Frankel, & Meyers, 1992). By using the same NELS survey item at the local level, LEA personnel would be able to compare how their schools respond to this benchmark value. Although there are technical problems with formal statistical comparisons to the national results, LEA staff can informally compare their results on the same survey questions to the results reported for the nation as a whole.

HOW DO I OBTAIN THIS INFORMATION?

To increase one's NIDSL, special services and other LEA personnel simply need to contact the appropriate federal office and ask to be placed on specific mailing lists. For the NCES data collection programs, one should first request a copy of the annual *Programs and Plans of the National Center for Education Statistics*. This is a very readable report that describes the major data collection activities of the NCES. It includes general descriptions of the major educational data collection programs of the NCES. After identifying those specific data collection programs (e.g., NELS, NALS, NAEP) that are of potential interest, an individual simply needs to contact NCES and indicate the specific data collection program mailing lists to which one wants to be added. Also, interested LEA personnel should request a copy of the Office of Educational Research and Improvement's (OERI) *Directory of Computer Data Files* and a copy of the NCEO's *Disability Summary Analyses of Select National Data Collection Programs* document (McGrew & Spiegel, 1993).

For similar information regarding the Department of Health and Human Services programs, an individual should request a copy of NCHS's *Catalog of Electronic Data Products, Catalog of Publications,* and a document called *Data Systems of the National Center for Health Statistics*. Finally, a request should be made for a document published by the *National Technical Information Service* (NTIS) entitled *A Directory of Federal Statistical Data Files*. Contact information for all of these documents is summarized in Table 4.

COMMENTS

LEA personnel are busy educating children and youth where the "rubber meets the road" in education. Although a parochial focus on local concerns and individual student needs and outcomes is understandable, a broader "big picture" perspective can improve an educator's ability to effectively make an impact at the local level. By becoming more familiar with national data collection programs, special services staff can: (a) better understand the multiple direct and indirect factors that influence the education of children and

TABLE 4. Select Agencies That Provide Information Regarding National
Data Collection Programs

Agency	Contact Information
National Center for Education Statistics (NCES)	Education Information Branch 555 New Jersey Ave. N. W. Washington, DC 20208
National Center for Health Statistics (NCHS)	6525 Belcrest Road Hyattsville, MD 20782
National Technical Information Services (NTIS)	5285 Port Royal Road Springfield, VA 22161
Office of Educational Research and Improvement (OERI)	Education Information Branch 555 New Jersey Ave., N. W. Washington, DC 20208
National Center for Education Outcomes (NCEO)	350 Elliott Hall 75 E. River Road University of Minnesota Minneapolis, MN 55455

youth, (b) better understand and participate in local, state, and national education reform discussions, and (c) develop local evaluation activities that produce more technically sound information that can be interpreted within a broader national context.

REFERENCES

Bronfenbrenner, U. (1979). *The ecology of human development: Experiments by nature and design.* Cambridge, MA: Harvard University Press.

Hanford, T., & White, K. (1991, June). Reform. *The American School Board, 178*(6), 14-16.

Ingels, S. J., Scott, L. A., Lindmark, J. T., Frankel, M. R., & Myers, S. L. (1992). *Users manual for National Education Longitudinal Study of 1988–First follow-up: Student component data file user's manual* (Vol 1). Washington, DC: U.S. Department of Education, Office of Educational Research and Improvement.

McGrew, K. S., & Spiegel, A. S. (1993). *Disability summary analyses of select national data collection programs.* Minneapolis, MN: National Center on Educational Outcomes, University of Minnesota.

McGrew, K. S., Spiegel, A. S., Thurlow, M. L., & Kim, D. (1994). *Matching information in national data collection programs to a model of school completion outcomes and indicators.* Minneapolis, MN: National Center on Educational Outcomes, University of Minnesota.

McGrew, K. S., Spiegel, A. S., Thurlow, M. L., Ysseldyke, J. E., Bruininks, R. H., & Shriner, J. G. (1992). *Outcomes for children and youth with disabilities: Secondary analysis of national data collection programs.* Minneapolis, MN: National Center on Educational Outcomes, University of Minnesota.

NCES. (1991). *Programs and plans of the National Center for Education Statistics: 1991 edition.* Washington, DC: National Center for Education Statistics.

Ysseldyke, J. E., Thurlow, M. L., Bruininks, R. H., Gilman, C. J., Deno, S. L., McGrew, K. S., & Shriner, J. G. (1992). *An evolving conceptual model of educational outcomes for children and youth with disabilities.* Minneapolis, MN: National Center for Educational Outcomes, University of Minnesota.

Opportunity-to-Learn Standards

James E. Ysseldyke
Martha L. Thurlow
Hyeonsook Shin

National Center on Educational Outcomes
University of Minnesota

SUMMARY. "Opportunity to learn" is a term that emerged in the vernacular of policymakers just within the past few years. Opportunity-to-learn (OTL) standards and their implications for students with disabilities need to be defined and examined carefully. Repeated calls for standards of excellence and greater accountability for results eventually have led to concerns about holding students responsible for reaching high academic standards when they have not had fair opportunities to learn. In this article, we discuss OTL standards, with special emphasis on alternative perspectives on OTL standards, primary positions advocated about OTL standards, and the implications of OTL standards for students with disabilities.

Repeated calls for standards of excellence and greater accountability for results have led to concerns about holding students accountable for reaching high academic standards when they have

---

The preparation of this article was supported in part through a cooperative agreement (H159C00004) with the U.S. Department of Education, Office of Special Education Programs. Points of view or opinions expressed in this article are not necessarily those of the Department of Education or offices within it.

Address correspondence to: James E. Ysseldyke, 350 Elliott Hall, 75 East River Road, University of Minnesota, Minneapolis, MN 55455.

[Haworth co-indexing entry note]: "Opportunity-to-Learn Standards." Ysseldyke, James, E., Martha L. Thurlow, and Hyeonsook Shin. Co-published simultaneously in *Special Services in the Schools* (The Haworth Press, Inc.) Vol. 9, No. 2, 1994, pp. 63-78; and: *Educational Outcomes for Students with Disabilities* (ed: James E. Ysseldyke, and Martha L. Thurlow) The Haworth Press, Inc., 1994, pp. 63-78. Multiple copies of this article/chapter may be purchased from The Haworth Document Delivery Center [1-800-3-HAWORTH; 9:00 a.m. - 5:00 p.m. (EST)].

not been provided the opportunity to learn. The notion of "opportunity-to-learn" standards is in the education reform legislation signed by President Clinton on March 31,1994. This legislation, known as "Goals 2000: Educate America Act" (PL 103-227), sets out eight national education goals, re-establishes the National Education Goals Panel to monitor progress toward goals, promotes the setting of high standards, establishes a national committee to oversee standards-setting efforts and approve state standards and assessments, encourages and supports state efforts around standards and assessments, and establishes national skill standards to define what workers need to know. Educational reform for students with disabilities also is addressed in Goals 2000. PL 103-277 is expected to "serve as a vehicle for making the promise of Part B of IDEA [the Individuals with Disabilities Education Act] a reality for all students with disabilities" (Kennedy, 1993, p. 20). Under Goals 2000, "students with disabilities . . . must be an integral part of all aspects of education reform, including the application of the National Education Goals and objectives, the establishment of national and state content, performance, and opportunity-to-learn standards" (Kennedy, 1993, p. 20). The language that accompanied the signed Senate version of Goals 2000 is informative. The Committee stated its expectation that Goals 2000 will serve "students with disabilities, including lesser known and newly emerging disabilities and students with significant and multiple disabilities . . . [in] all aspects of educational reform, including . . . opportunity-to-learn standards" (Kennedy, 1993, p. 20).

In this article, we discuss "opportunity-to-learn" (OTL) standards, alternative perspectives on OTL standards, and primary positions advocated about OTL standards. Concerns about students with disabilities are treated in discussions of OTL standards, current proposals regarding the measurement of OTL, and major issues surrounding the concept of OTL. We conclude with a discussion of the implications of OTL standards for students with disabilities and related services personnel who work with these students.

PERSPECTIVES ON OTL STANDARDS

Although opportunity-to-learn (OTL) standards emerged from the national debate over national standards and testing, the term has been defined and used in different ways by different groups. Some groups use the terms OTL and school delivery standards interchangeably, while others extend the notion of OTL standards to include a wide range of criteria to be used for system-wide educational reform. Other groups that differentiate OTL standards from school delivery standards emphasize some components of schooling such as curriculum and instruction, resources, and inputs. Traiman's (1993) five different ways to define "opportunity to learn" represent the diverse perspectives that exist on the OTL standards. According to Traiman, opportunity to learn should be parsimonious and limited to criteria that are directly related to the provision of high quality curriculum and instruction based on challenging academic standards, and include other critical factors deemed essential to quality teaching and learning, including safe and drug-free schools and indicators of effective schools and professional practice. OTL standards also should include all systemic changes needed for students to succeed, information on what actions a state will take if students fail to meet established performance standards, and provide measures of the adequacy of funding available at each school.

The main perspectives that continue to characterize discussions of OTL standards include (a) OTL as equivalent to school delivery standards, (b) OTL as part of systemic reform, (c) OTL as sufficient inputs, and (d) OTL as allocated or academic engaged time. Each of these is discussed briefly here.

OTL standards as equivalent to school delivery standards. One perspective is that opportunity to learn standards are the same as school delivery standards. Traiman and Goren (1993) noted that "school delivery standards are now referred to as opportunity-to-learn standards" (p. 6), and that their purpose is to protect students from being unfairly held responsible for failing to reach the content and performance standards when they have not had the opportunity to learn the material in the content standards.

Andrew Porter (1993a), who directs the Center for Education Research at the University of Wisconsin and has written extensively on opportunity-to-learn standards, referred to and quoted the meaning of school delivery standards that was used in the 1992 House Bill on restructuring schools: "School delivery standards means the standards necessary to ensure that each student in a school has a fair opportunity to achieve the knowledge and skills set out in the National Content Standards and Work-force Readiness Standards" (quoted by Porter, 1993a, p. 2). In the discussion of school delivery standards, Porter (1993b) differentiated school delivery standards from opportunity-to-learn standards, although he recognized that two terms are being used interchangeably. Porter defined opportunity-to-learn standards as "the enacted curriculum as experienced by the student" (Porter, 1993b, p. 7). Even though Porter expanded the coverage of opportunity-to-learn standards from just the content of instruction to "the pedagogical quality of instruction and the resources that are available to students and teachers" (Porter, 1993b, p. 7), he also pointed out that opportunity-to-learn standards are less inclusive than school delivery standards in that opportunity-to-learn standards do not address school organizational characteristics and drug-free safe school environments. However, according to Porter (1993b), school delivery standards include not only opportunity to learn but also quality of school life factors.

OTL standards as part of systemic reform. At a 1992 meeting sponsored by the National Governors' Association, participants suggested that OTL standards be used in a variety of ways, "depending on whether they focus on inputs (e.g., teacher training, provision of appropriate textbooks), processes (e.g., instruction), outcomes (e.g., student performance), or a combination of all" (Traiman & Goren, 1993, p. 6). Traiman and Goren (1993) also identified a key issue in determining the degree of specificity and the intended use of the OTL standards. Should OTL standards include all systemic changes needed for all students to succeed or be limited to a few criteria directly related to the provision of high-quality curriculum and instruction? In discussions of systemic educational reform, OTL standards address the quality and availability of curriculum, materials, and technologies; teacher training and professional development; provision of a safe and secure environment for learning; provision of resources such as libraries and laboratories or other related services; and aligned policies on curriculum, instruction, and assessment.

OTL standards as sufficient inputs. For some, students are considered to have the opportunity to learn as long as schools allocate resources to instruction and fund programs. Educational inputs and resources are considered necessary for improving student achievement. The National Council on Education Standards and Testing (1992) identified input conditions that are fundamental to providing all children with the opportunity to learn. These conditions include, but are not limited to, "teachers who are trained to teach the content of the content standards, appropriate and high-quality instructional materials which reflect the content standards, and curriculum that covers the material of the content standards in sufficient scope and with adequate sequence for students to master it to high performance standards" (National Council on Education Standards and Testing, 1992, p. E-5). Content and instructional quality are viewed by Porter (1993b) as the two best predictors of student achievement and as the essence of the OTL standards.

The current discussion about opportunity-to-learn standards proposes that assuring that all students have equal opportunity to reach ambitious outcomes requires not only equal access to inputs but also effective use of inputs/resources at school (Fuhrman & Elmore, 1993). One of several approaches to the effective use of resources is to create professional standards or incentives for more effective use of resources. More emphasis may be placed on professional development and teacher preparation to encourage good practice in the effective use of resources. For instance, teacher education and professional development (new Goal 4) and parent involvement (new Goal 8) were added as national education goals in Goals 2000.

OTL as allocated time or academic engaged time. Time is a recurring notion to people who are concerned about the teaching-learning process in classroom settings. Speaking on behalf of the Commission on Chapter 1, Haycock (1993) mentioned "time" in addition to other commonly identified variables, as a variable for helping students reach high performance standards. According to Haycock's testimony, states must determine whether schools provide extra time for students who need it, in addition to time during the regular schedule for teachers to assess students' progress, meet with parents, and learn how to improve their own skills. This notion is reinforced by recent policy documents that stress time as a key part of the opportunity a student has to learn (Anderson & Walberg, 1993; Moore & Funkhouser, 1990; National Education Commission on Time and Learning, 1994). Another example is the conclusions of *A Nation at Risk* (National Commission on Excellence in Education, 1983), which discussed insufficient time devoted to instruction. Initial reactions to this focused on extending the school year and extending the length of the school day. Following this, conceptualizations of time were refined, and positive relationships shown between time allocated to instruction, engaged time, and student achievement (Cooley & Leinhardt, 1980; Denham & Lieberman, 1980; Stanley & Greenwood, 1983; Thurlow, Graden, Greener, & Ysseldyke, 1983; Ysseldyke, Christenson, Thurlow, & Skiba, 1987).

The concept of time spent in learning has been called "Academic Learning Time" (ALT) by the Beginning Teacher Evaluation Study (BTES) researchers. ALT is an engaged time variable that includes only the time during which the student is engaged in a task that can be performed with high success. Gettinger (1984, 1985) presented the notion of time needed for learning, noting that students differ in the amount of time they need to reach a certain criterion of mastery. Thus, time spent or time allocated relates inconsistently to learning when the amount of time needed is not taken into account. Concern about time needed for learning represents the argument that there needs to be fair and sufficient opportunity to learn.

WHAT ARE PEOPLE ADVOCATING FOR OTL STANDARDS?

Prior to the passage of Goals 2000, people were taking various positions on the importance and need for OTL standards. Although the passed legislation retained OTL standards in a voluntary way, among the main positions were ones that argued to (a) not include these types of standards in Goals 2000, (b) mandate OTL standards, and (c) keep OTL standards voluntary. Review of these positions provides additional information about the OTL concept.

Do not include OTL standards in Goals 2000. Opponents of a federal role in the development and implementation of OTL standards were fearful about including the OTL standards in federal legislation because they thought it was too difficult to define OTL standards, because it would be too hard to measure, or because it would result in chaos to try to implement OTL standards. They expressed concerns over the unintended infringement on states' and local education agencies' constitutional responsibility for education practices and policy. Traiman and Goren (1993) also identified the apprehension that "OTL standards will be much too prescriptive, require burdensome documentation, and inhibit local creativity" (p. 7).

First, there was not an agreed-upon definition of what constitutes fair opportunity. OTL standards were being defined differently by different people, depending on their viewpoint about the degree of specificity or the intended use of the standards. Thus, a concern was raised about whether the hard-to-define OTL standards should be included in federal legislation. OTL standards were even regarded as "the riskiest part of Goals 2000" (Barth, 1993, p. 3). Second, it also was argued that OTL standards should not be included in federal legislation because they are too hard to measure. Such a concern was about what, how, and when to measure in order to know whether students had opportunities to learn. One of the concerns was that OTL standards should not be a mere checklist of inputs, resources, and curriculum content areas (Crandall, 1993). Another concern was whether the measurement of OTL standards should be delayed until outcome measures signal a problem, rather than measuring all schools (Traiman & Goren, 1993). Third, it was very likely that different places would go about developing and implementing opportunity-to-learn standards in many different ways. It was seen as very likely that the lack of clarity would, in turn, lead to confusion and chaos over a number of legal issues that would dramatically increase the likelihood of lawsuits on the failure to provide sufficient opportunity to learn.

Mandate OTL standards. The federal role in the development and implementation of OTL standards has been controversial. The rationale behind wanting the mandatory standards was that students should be held responsible for learning challenging content only if they had appropriate opportunities to learn. The federal government may be charged with both identifying state and local policies and practices that foster opportunity to learn and making every effort to distribute federal resources equitably to disadvantaged students and students with special needs who are most in need of support to achieve high national content and performance standards (Traiman & Goren, 1993).

Many proponents of OTL standards claimed that the standards should not be so highly prescriptive (Porter, 1993a) or excessively inclusive that they would stifle local flexibility (Darling-Hammond, 1993). Lehman (1993) dismissed the concerns that OTL standards tend to be too prescriptive, arguing that they should be mandatory in order to support, or put pressure on, school districts in which many students are not achieving at the expected level.

Keep OTL standards voluntary. A report by the National Governors' Association (NGA) stated that "the Governors strongly affirm that states, not the federal government, should assume the responsibility for creating an education delivery system that enables all students to achieve high standards" (NGA, 1992-1993, p. 2; also cited by Olson, 1993, p. 32). According to this statement, the development and use of OTL standards should be each state's responsibility and should not be mandated through federal legislation. Each state would be allowed to develop its own OTL standards to meet the educational goals of the state.

HOW ARE STUDENTS WITH DISABILITIES TREATED IN DISCUSSIONS OF OTL STANDARDS?

Students with disabilities are treated in multiple ways in the discussion of OTL standards. The range goes from no mention of students with disabilities to special emphasis on them. Future discussions may even suggest different types of OTL for different groups of students (for more information on future issues, see Ysseldyke, Thurlow, & Geenen, this volume).

Students with disabilities are not mentioned. OTL standards address concerns about the possibility that the consequences of inadequacies and inequities in curriculum, instruction and learning environments are unfairly imputed to students rather than to schools and school systems. Much attention seems to have been paid to poor and minority students; however, those students with disabilities who have not had enough opportunities to learn the content reflected in outcome measures are scarcely mentioned in the argument for OTL standards.

Extensive attention given to students with disabilities. Some people suggest that students with disabilities should get much more opportunity to learn than students without disabilities. Such a concern seems to have been raised by proponents of a federal role in protecting and providing educational opportunities to children with disabilities as well as disadvantaged children (Traiman & Goren, 1993).

Carnine (undated) raised the issues of *how* those students with disabilities and those in poverty will learn what they should learn. Rather than reducing expectations for the achievement of students with disabilities, providing those students with access to quality education can be one of the ways to help them attain high expectations reflected in challenging curriculum standards. Carnine (undated) identified the quality educational tools that are particularly critical for lower-performing students. Those educational tools include explicit learning strategy instruction, instructional guidance and supports, relevant prior knowledge, and appropriately varied review.

HOW DO PEOPLE PROPOSE TO MEASURE OTL?

Just as conceptions of opportunity to learn vary considerably from one person to the next, or one organization to the next, so do conceptions of how OTL should be measured. For some, opportunity to learn is best reflected by the amount of *time spent in school.* They advocate lengthening the school day or the school year as ways to increase opportunity to learn. Several researchers suggest that the amount of *time allocated to instruction* be measured as an index of OTL because a considerable amount of time spent in school could be spent in non-instructional activities. Minutes or hours allocated to instruction is one way to measure allocated time. Another way is to count the number of hours of academic content that students take, or to count credit hours delivered. However, time spent in school and time allocated to instruction may be inadequate indices of opportunity to learn because during those times students still may not be actively engaged in responding to instruction. Thus, some propose measuring *academic engaged time, active learning time* or *active responding time* as an index of OTL. The methodology used to measure the amount of engaged time usually consists of observing in classrooms and counting (usually using an interval recording method) the number of intervals in which students are actively engaged. Greenwood (1991) and Ysseldyke and associates (e.g., Ysseldyke, Thurlow, Mecklenburg, & Graden, 1984), for example, used the Code for Instructional Structure and Student Academic Response (CISSAR). Greenwood (1993) has now developed the Ecobehavioral Assessment Software System (EBASS) to be used in gathering data on student active responding, inappropriate behavior, and task management responses. For others, opportunity to learn is best measured by counting the amount of *money spent* on the provision of instruction. Indices of money spent could be the overall school budget, per pupil expenditure, or teacher salaries.

Measuring opportunity to learn using teacher logs provides information on the *coverage of the enacted curriculum* as experienced by the student. As Porter indicated (1993a, 1993b), teacher interviews or daily logs can be used to measure how well OTL standards are being met. Porter (1993b) also presented content taxonomies in science and math as a framework that a teacher can rely on when indicating the content of instruction and instructional practices for each day of instruction for an entire school year. Content coverage is indicated by topics covered in the class period and the amount of emphasis placed on the topic. Teachers are also asked to indicate the modes of instruction, the types of activities students engaged in, and instructional materials used (Porter, 1993b).

MAJOR ISSUES

Several major issues surround the notion of opportunity-to-learn standards. Many of these issues, either directly or indirectly, are related to the implementation of standards and their incorporation within current state policies and practices. First, there are significant disagreements about the *definition of opportunity to learn.* Obviously, if OTL is defined differently in different settings, then indices of OTL in different settings, districts, or states cannot be compared.

Second, the process of *measuring* how well each school is meeting the standards per se runs the risk of transforming the standards into checklists of minimum amounts or types of resources and practices. This would spoil the rationale behind the setting of such standards. Billings (1993) also mentioned the need to measure OTL standards "by means of a carefully designed school accreditation process. After a careful self-analysis, a visiting team of accreditors could determine the levels at which the standards are being met and recommend any needed steps for improvement" (p. 2).

Third, there is controversy over whether OTL standards can or should be used for *accountability purposes.* In contrast to Porter's argument (1993a) that school delivery standards should not be used for accountability, Darling-Hammond (1993) argued in favor of the use of OTL standards as "a critical component of an accountability system" (p. 1). Attention should be paid to "resources and learning experiences required for students to achieve the intellectually and practically challenging learning outcomes envisioned by current school reform initiatives" (Darling-Hammond, 1993, p. 1). The use of data on educational outcomes (e.g., test scores, graduation rates, drop-out rates) as a sole basis for assessing school quality has provided distorted information on school practices in distributing equitable access to educational opportunities and, further, may result in the exclusion of students from disadvantaged backgrounds in order to maintain a good image via student performance levels. Exclusion could be accomplished by retaining low-performing students in grade, placing them in special education programs, or letting them drop out (Allington & McGill-Franzen, 1992). Improvements in educational resources and processes might be targeted to increase student achievement and guarantee accountable schools, in order to avoid any attempt to limit enrollment or participation of low-performing students in school programs as a way to produce apparently good outcomes (Darling-Hammond, 1992).

Fourth, if, as is assumed in school reform, all children can learn challenging content and complex problem solving skills, "*dumbing down* the material for the disadvantaged represents a clear denial of their opportunity to learn challenging material of the curriculum" (O'Day & Smith, 1993, p. 264). OTL standards should not refer to minimum standards encompassed in notions of a basic skills curriculum, minimum competency tests and compensatory education.

Fifth, there are different perspectives on *when OTL standards should be applied* since OTL standards, by definition, involve many different components of the educational system and measurement of these components necessarily will take time and resources. One perspective is that we should not worry about measuring OTL until we have outcomes information that signals a problem (D. W. Hornbeck, personal communication, Dec. 3, 1993). Another perspective is that both opportunity to learn and outcomes should be measured at the same time. For instance, participants in the 1992 NGA meeting claimed that OTL standards involve both outcomes and inputs/processes (Traiman & Goren, 1993).

Sixth, we currently have *state policies* for the accreditation of schools as well as procedures for the review of school quality. For instance, Kansas supports a process of accreditation as a statewide monitoring system, which is called the Kansas Quality Performance Accreditation (Swall & Finley, 1993). To some minimal extent, the basic OTL notion is already incorporated within these existing mechanisms. However, they could be incorporated to a much greater extent. The inclusion of the opportunity-to-learn notion within federal education reform law will be a first step toward greater incorporation of OTL standards into state policies and school review practices.

IMPLICATIONS FOR STUDENTS WITH DISABILITIES

In *Raising Standards for American Education,* the National Council on Education Standards and Testing (1992) noted that "if not accompanied by measures to ensure equal opportunity to learn, national content and performance standards could help widen the achievement gap between the advantaged and the disadvantaged in our society" (p. E-12). This is a basic equity issue that continues to be discussed. However, there are several other implications that OTL standards have for students with disabilities.

First, there is a historical tendency in our country to exclude students with disabilities from discussions of assessment and accountability-related issues. These students often are forgotten in discussions of OTL standards. If students with disabilities are not included in measurements of OTL, then there is the distinct risk that they will be viewed as unimportant, second-class citizens. If policy decisions are made using data on only a portion of the school-age population, then there is a risk of inaccurate policy decision making.

Second, there is a significant *cost* involved in providing special education services to students with disabilities. In general, students with disabilities need more equipment, lower student-teacher ratios, and a number of other costly provisions. If some index of *funding* is used as the measure of OTL, then students with disabilities are going to appear to receive much more opportunity to learn than many other students. No one to our knowledge has talked about balancing a funding measure with resources needed.

Third, there is little discussion of the *qualitative nature of instruction* when talking about OTL. Ysseldyke and Christenson (1993) contend that the qualitative nature of instruction for two students can be very different in the same classroom at the same time when taught by the same teacher using the same teaching tactics. Ysseldyke and Christenson advocate formal measurement of the student's instructional needs in the context of classroom and home environments.

Fourth, a question is posed as to whether we have to provide *comparable or necessary* opportunities to learn for students with disabilities. Should low functioning students get the same amount of time as everybody else or the amount of time necessary for them to be successful? This question makes the distinction between absolute measures of opportunity to learn and measures that are weighted in some way by the need exhibited by the student. For instance, Spady (1994), in advocating outcome-based education, argued that the goals of instruction should remain constant across students, but that time to learn might vary.

CONCLUSIONS AND RECOMMENDATIONS

Developing reasonable and fair opportunity-to-learn standards is a challenge, particularly when students with disabilities are considered. Despite arguments for and against these kinds of standards, it is difficult to leave them out of the picture when students are required to reach high academic standards.

Given that opportunity to learn is an important part of achieving high academic standards, it is important to recommend the nature of these standards. In the final version of Goals 2000, it was made clear that those defining opportunity to learn must consider: curricula, instructional materials, and technologies; teacher capabilities; professional development for teachers, principals, and administrators; alignment of curriculum, instructional practices, and assessments with content standards; safety and security of the learning environment; availability of resources for learning and instruction, such as libraries and laboratories; policies, curricula and instructional practices that ensure non-discrimination on the basis of gender; and other factors that help ensure that students receive a fair opportunity to achieve the knowledge and skills in the content performance standards (Goals 2000: Educate America Act of 1994, § 213(c)(2)). These factors, of course, are relatively limited in their coverage. However, viewing opportunity to learn as something more than just the financial resources in a school is noteworthy.

It will be critical that the development of OTL standards involve all communities that will be affected by the Goals 2000 legislation. Of particular concern, here, of course is the involvement of individuals with disabilities or of individuals familiar with disability issues. This currently is a requirement of the law for the formation of the Council that will certify voluntary national standards including OTL standards. How this requirement will be played out when the Council (called the National Education Standards and Improvement Council) is formed will be of interest to many.

Another important recommendation is that the effects of the legislation on students with disabilities be monitored. Again, this is a provision included in the final legislation. Either the National Academy of Sciences or the National Academy of Education will conduct an analysis of the extent to which students with disabilities are included in (or, excluded from) Goals 2000 reform activities.

REFERENCES

Allington, R., & McGill-Franzen, A. (1992). Unintended effects of educational reform in New York. *Educational Policy, 6*(4), 397-414.
Anderson, L. W., & Walberg, H. J. (Ed.) (1993). *Timepiece: Extending and enhancing learning time.* Reston, VA: National Association of Secondary School Principals.
Barth, P. (1993). Clinton's Goals 2000. *Basic Education, 37*(10), 1-4.
Billings, J. A. (1993). *Summary of Written Testimony Submitted to NGA on*

Opportunity-To-Learn Standards. Washington, DC: National Governors' Association.

Carnine, D. (undated). *Opportunity to learn standards: Design features of quality educational tools.* Eugene, OR: University of Oregon.

Cooley, W., & Leinhardt, G. (1980). The instructional dimensions study. *Educational Evaluation and Policy Analysis, 2,* 7-24.

Crandall, D. P. (1993). *Summary of Written Testimony Submitted to NGA on Opportunity-To-Learn Standards.* Washington, DC: National Governors' Association.

Darling-Hammond, L. (1992). *Standards of Practice for Learner-Centered Schools* (Commissioned Paper). Albany, NY: State Department of Education.

Darling-Hammond, L. (1993). *Summary of Written Testimony Submitted to NGA on Opportunity-To-Learn Standards.* Washington, DC: National Governors' Association.

Denham, C., & Lieberman, A. (Eds.). (1980). *Time to Learn.* Washington, DC: National Institute of Education.

Fuhrman, S. H., & Elmore, R. F. (1993). *Opportunity to learn and the state role: An outline for a paper.* New Brunswick, NJ: Center for Policy Research in Education.

Gettinger, M. (1984). Individual differences in time needed for learning: A review of literature. *Educational Psychologist, 19*(1), 15-29.

Gettinger, M. (1985). Time allocated and time spent relative to time needed for learning as determinants of achievement. *Journal of Educational Psychology, 77*(1), 3-11.

Greenwood, C. (1991). Longitudinal analyses of time, engagement, and achievement in at-risk versus non-risk students. *Exceptional Children, 57*(6), 521-535.

Greenwood, C. (1993). *Ecobehavioral assessment software system (EBASS).* Kansas City, KS: Juniper Gardens Children's Project.

Haycock, K. (1993). *Summary of Written Testimony Submitted to NGA on Opportunity-To-Learn Standards.* Washington, DC: National Governors' Association.

Kennedy, R. (1993). *Goals 2000: Educate America Act.: Report together with additional and minority views.* Congress Report from the Committee on Labor and Human Resources. Calendar No. 106. 103D Congress 1st Session. Report 103-85.

Lehman, P. R. (1993). Summary of Written Testimony Submitted to NGA on Opportunity-To-Learn Standards. Washington, DC: National Governors' Association.

Moore, M. T., & Funkhouser, J. (1990). *More time to learn: Extended time strategies for Chapter 1 students.* Washington, DC: Decision Resources Corporation.

National Commission on Excellence in Education. (1983). *A nation at risk: The imperative for educational reform.* Washington, DC: U.S. Government Printing Office.

National Council on Education Standards and Testing. (1992). *Raising standards for American Education.* Washington, D.C.: U.S. Government Printing Office.

National Education Commission on Time and Learning. (1994). *Prisoners of time.* Washington, DC: U.S. Government Printing Office.

NGA. (1992-1993). *Providing an opportunity to learn: Principles for states.* Washington, DC: National Governors' Association Task Force on Education.

O'Day, J. A., & Smith, M. S. (1993). Systemic reform and educational opportunity. In S. Fuhrman (Ed.), *Designing coherent policy: Improving the system.* San Francisco, CA: Jossey Bass.

Olson, L. (1993). N.G.A. offering states advice on 'opportunity' standards. *Education Week, 8*(1), 32.

Porter, A. C. (1993a). School delivery standards. *Educational Researcher, 14*(4), 24-30.

Porter, A. C. (1993b). *Defining and measuring opportunity to learn.* Madison, WI: University of Wisconsin.

Spady, W. G. (1994). Choosing outcomes of significance. *Educational Leadership, 51*(6), 18-22.

Stanley, S. O., & Greenwood, C. R. (1983). How much "opportunity to respond" does the minority, disadvantaged student receive in school? *Exceptional Children, 49,* 370-373.

Swall, R., & Finley, S. (1993). *Quality performance accreditation in special education: An annotated bibliography.* Lawrence, KS: The University of Kansas.

Thurlow, M. L., Graden, J., Greener, J. W., & Ysseldyke, J. E. (1983). LD and non-LD students' opportunities to learn. *Learning Disability Quarterly, 6,* 172-183.

Traiman, S. (1993). *The debate on opportunity-to-learn standards.* Washington, DC: National Governor's Association.

Traiman, S., & Goren, P. (1993). Understanding opportunity to learn. *Basic Education, 37*(10), 5-9.

Ysseldyke, J. E., & Christenson, S. L. (1993). *The instructional environment system–II.* Longmont, CO: Sopris West.

Ysseldyke, J. E., Christenson, S. L., Thurlow, M. L., & Skiba, R. (1987). *Academic engagement and active responding of mentally retarded, learning disabled, emotionally disturbed and nonhandicapped elementary students* (Research Report 4). Minneapolis, MN: University of Minnesota, Instructional Alternatives Project.

Ysseldyke, J. E., Thurlow, M. L., Mecklenburg, C., & Graden, J. (1984). Opportunity to learn for regular and special education students during reading instruction. *Remedial and Special Education, 5*(1), 29-37.

What Is OBE and What Does It Mean for Students with Disabilities?

Carol B. Massanari

Mid-South Regional Resource Center
University of Kentucky

SUMMARY. Outcome-based education (OBE) is a vehicle for changing from an emphasis on educational process to an emphasis on the outcomes of education. Unfortunately, it is a term that has been surrounded by misunderstanding, confusion and resistance. This article discusses and clarifies the term OBE. In addition, a model for using the term "outcome" is proposed and illustrations of how the term could be used at all levels of the education system are provided.

Bud could not wait to leave school. There was no way he was going to stay past the designated 12 years even though he had the option to stay until 21. So he went through graduation and picked up his diploma just like everyone else. At 33 he still was living at home. The feed mill where he spent his days doing odd jobs for a nominal wage shut down. He had been given "work" at the mill originally because it was owned by a friend of the family; and he stayed on as new owners took over. Now with the mill closed, he had no work and no skills.

Address correspondence to: Carol B. Massanari, Mid-South Regional Resource Center, 114 Mineral Industries Building, Lexington, KY 40506-0051.

[Haworth co-indexing entry note]: "What Is OBE and What Does It Mean for Students with Disabilities?" Massanari, Carol B. Co-published simultaneously in *Special Services in the Schools* (The Haworth Press, Inc.) Vol. 9, No. 2, 1994, pp. 79-92; and: *Educational Outcomes for Students with Disabilities* (ed: James E. Ysseldyke, and Martha L. Thurlow) The Haworth Press, Inc., 1994, pp. 79-92. Multiple copies of this article/chapter may be purchased from The Haworth Document Delivery Center [1-800-3-HAWORTH; 9:00 a.m. - 5:00 p.m. (EST)].

Even though he had received a diploma, Bud had no academic skills to speak of, few self-help skills and no vocational skills. Literally, Bud received a diploma, not because he had learned anything in school, but because he had attended school faithfully for the designated number of days and hours. He had done quite well completing the required amount of "seat time." But that seat time requirement did nothing to help him become a functional or independent adult.

How many Buds are there and how many more Buds will it take to force us to change our focus from process to outcome? Sure Bud might be an extreme illustration and it can be argued that he simply missed out on the advantages of P.L. 94-142, but unfortunately, the data from follow-up studies have been telling us that too many students with disabilities are not finding work and are not living independently after leaving school (Wagner et al., 1991). While there may be many variables that help explain this situation, a primary variable is the education that students receive while in school. In an effort to improve this variable, recent and current efforts are focusing on the need to improve education by focusing on desired results, i.e., outcomes.

Bud illustrates what can happen when we are more concerned with process than results. The main criteria for Bud to receive a diploma was the completion of 12 years in school for a designated number of days (i.e., seat time criteria). Being concerned with the amount of time a student spends in school is one example of process criteria. Other examples of process include having a completed IEP that meets regulatory standards or having completed a course of studies with a passing grade. Unfortunately, a well-written IEP or a passing grade (in many instances 60% to 70% is passing) do not indicate that a student has acquired the skills needed to perform real life functions.

The movement toward an outcome-based education (OBE) has grown from a desire to change our focus on process criteria to a focus on results criteria. OBE forces us to look at what we want students to be able to do as a result of having spent time in school. If Bud had attended a school that operated under an OBE philosophy, he would have been required to demonstrate that he had learned and could apply specific skills before graduating or receiving a diploma. If Bud's education had centered around real-life skill acquisition, perhaps he would not have been so anxious to leave school, and perhaps he would have been living independently with a full-time job at age 33.

Even though this may sound reasonable enough, there is a great deal of resistance, confusion and misunderstanding about OBE. This article attempts to provide some clarification by providing one perspective of the definition of OBE, proposing a model for using the term "outcome," and illustrating the use of outcomes at all levels of the education system.

THE ESSENCE OF OBE

At the heart of outcome-based education is the belief that all aspects of education must be focused on the desired end product, the result. In order to determine the necessary interventions, one must first know where one wants to finish. It is a process that requires determining the desired results and then working backward to determine the skills and knowledge needed to achieve those results.

OBE means basing decisions about instruction, curriculum, assessment, school structure and other aspects of education on the results we want to achieve. Integral to this process is the belief that all children can learn well that which is taught well. A set of expected results and shared beliefs about education are the beginning steps of educational change. There are a minimum of four critical steps to OBE: (1) determine the desired results and articulate beliefs about education; (2) identify proven effective strategies for achieving the results and acting in accordance with beliefs; (3) implement changes to align practice with desired results and proven effective strategies; and (4) continuously assess and make adjustments.

OBE is not a prescribed product, curriculum, textbook, intervention strategy, monitoring tool or testing program. Many confuse OBE with Mastery Learning, an approach to improve instruction developed by Benjamin Bloom based on the work of John Carroll (Cohen & Hyman, 1993; Glatthorn, 1993; O'Neil, 1993). While the development of Mastery Learning may have been a catalyst for

OBE and the two share a similar set of beliefs, Mastery Learning more precisely is an instructional process used in the classroom to help assure that students do achieve the predetermined, desired results. Because of the compatibility of Mastery Learning with OBE, many times Mastery Learning is used as one of the effective tools for improving instruction and changing teacher practice. However, it is important to remember that Master Learning is not, in and of itself, OBE. Neither are other products or curricular programs such as Brolin's (1989) Life-centered Career Education, in and of themselves, OBE. Rather, they are tools teachers can use in the instructional process that is part of OBE.

OBE is not concerned with how much time a student spends on a subject. Rather, OBE is concerned with whether a student can demonstrate that which the student is expected to learn. Traditional education is concerned with units of time and assuring that students spend enough time on a given subject area (e.g., the Carnegie Unit). Traditionally, a student moves on to the next subject, grade or unit when the time period is completed (e.g., a school year, a semester) and if the student has received a passing grade (e.g., anything above a D or 60% averaged from various assignments and tests over the designated period of time). OBE is concerned with whether a student can demonstrate that learning has taken place commensurate with a preset high level of expectation.

Finally, OBE does not promote failure or blame non-learning entirely on circumstances or students themselves. Certainly, students must be willing participants for learning to take place. But OBE forces educators to approach each situation with a belief that each child can learn and that the first responsibility of educators is to modify instruction based on that belief, on desired results and that which has proven to be effective practice. It is not acceptable to assume children cannot learn just because they come from a "poor" home environment or that failure resulting from incomplete assignments is *only* due to the student's own lack of motivation. Rather, it is important to continually and comprehensively evaluate all aspects of non-learning situations, including instructional approach, environment and student motivation.

CLARIFYING THE TERM OUTCOME

Defining the term "outcome" seems simple enough. A number of definitions have been proposed (DeStefano & Wagner, 1990; Shavelson, McDonnell & Oakes, 1989; Spady, 1992a, 1994; Ysseldyke et al. 1992). Regardless of how elaborate the definition, the bottom line is that outcome is equated with result. However, generating definitions appears simpler than using the term consistently, particularly when attempting to identify examples or indicators of outcomes. Examples and indicators differ depending on the individual's focus of concern.

Differences sometimes exist in the way that special educators and general educators identify outcomes. Differences sometimes exist between teacher-identified indicators of outcomes and those identified by state education (SEA) staff. Differences sometimes exist in what parents identify as outcomes and what those working at the national level or those involved in the political process identify as outcomes. And, those interested in accountability data might identify yet another set of outcomes.

While many of these differences are subtle, it is important to understand and clarify them if outcomes are to be used as the base for making educational decisions. One way of clarifying differences is to identify how the term is used and to begin using terms linked to the intended application. Three applications are addressed here.

Learning outcomes. A primary use of the term "outcome" refers to expectations set for students, competencies, skills and knowledge that students are expected to demonstrate as a result of learning. In this application, the term "outcomes" is used in two ways. First, there are *exit outcomes*, which are demonstrations of learning that take place at the completion of a period of learning activity (e.g., upon exit from school program, or grade; upon completion of a unit of study) (Spady, 1992a). Second, there are outcomes that are called *enabling outcomes*. These emerge when exit outcomes are broken into sets of skills and learning is individualized to meet different kinds of student needs (e.g., reading requirements, math skills, use of Braille, as well as dressing, mobility and social skills). Frey, Lynch, and Jakwerth (1991) have systematically identified sets of unique skills needed by students with varying disabilities in order for them to achieve the general expectations of schooling and assume adult roles. Most (if not all) of these skills, which are considered by many to be necessary outcomes for students with disabilities, are examples of outcomes that fit into this category of enabling outcomes. They are enabling because they are critical to the student's ability to achieve the broader exit outcomes. Whether exit or enabling, however, all of these outcomes are specifically associated with students in that students are expected to demonstrate the outcomes as a result of learning.

Actualized outcomes. Another use of the term "outcome" is in reference to the real-life experiences that students have after leaving school. These are the outcomes that have been identified through the transition and follow-along studies (Chadsey-Rusch, Rusch, & O'Reilly, 1991). They are the actualization of learning through the acquisition of a job, independent living and self-supporting income. These signify the actual use of skills after the formal learning period ends. While they involve the learner, the reported results may be influenced by factors outside the learner. These are the effects of juxtaposing the learning with the larger social system. For example, actualized outcome data related to employment might be influenced by available employment opportunities or available supports more than the individual's skills.

System outcomes. A third way in which outcome is used is to identify the extent to which the system generally is achieving desired results. These results are not direct evidence that the desired student learning has been achieved, yet they are critical to supporting and sustaining the learning, and are considered correlates of success in education. For example, if students are attending school and not dropping out, then we can presume that the system is achieving a desired expectation of motivating students to stay in school. Staying in school is not evidence that students are learning, yet being in school (at least for the present time) is a prerequisite if a student is to have the opportunity to learn the expected skills. Likewise, for students with disabilities, participation in an integrated setting is important to learning skills needed to demonstrate some expected learning outcomes. Other examples are found in family related issues, such as assuring that students arrive at school fed and healthy, and thus more ready to learn. Community related examples include the level of satisfaction and the willingness to support education.

Increasing attention is being given to system expectations as the debate about school delivery and opportunity-to-learn standards increases (Capitol Publications, 1993; National Governors' Association, 1993; see Ysseldyke, Thurlow, & Shin in this volume). Darling-Hammond (1992) proposed 12 standards to be considered when constructing an accountability system to support schools and student learning. All 12 standards could be developed into outcome statements and applied as system outcomes. Examples include statements such as "teachers demonstrate effective instructional skills" or "schools receive equitable funding." While these outcome expectations for the system alone do not guarantee the end result (e.g., young adults with real-life skills), they are critical to supporting and ensuring that the end product is attainable for all students.

APPLYING THE OBE PROCESS THROUGHOUT THE EDUCATION SYSTEM

OBE started as a means for influencing and changing the instructional process that occurs within classrooms. It was intended to change instructional practice by refocusing attention on the desired results of a defined unit of learning (e.g., end of school, end of year, end of content unit). Essentially, OBE started as an approach for improving decisions that have an impact on instruction at the local education level (i.e., the classroom, school building and district).

As the OBE movement has grown, it has expanded to include a larger context. Policy makers and others at state and national levels have adopted the OBE label and now appear to refer to OBE, not as a process of change for the local level only, but as a potential framework for transforming the entire education system. Within this expanded OBE framework, decisions about education would be made on the basis of desired and acquired outcomes, or end results. In other words, we would have an outcome-driven system of education.

Spady (1992b) indicated that OBE is driven by the need to re-focus and re-define the system, including the system's fundamental purposes, premises, principles and parameters. The process of re-focus and re-definition need not be limited to decisions at the local level. Rather, it provides significant potential for radically changing the perception, understanding and description of the education of students at all levels of the education system. The challenge lies in determining what outcomes are critical for meeting the various decision needs of the different levels of the system. When we have clearly identified the various outcomes that are important, information (hereafter referred to as data) about these outcomes can be used to meet the various responsibilities of each level of the education system.

National level. While a great emphasis is placed on education by many national politicians, education is, in fact, constitutionally a state responsibility. In the national arena, education-related actions have been taken to support and sustain the efforts of states to ensure a high quality of life for *all* citizens. In the end, the goal is to ensure the economic competitiveness of the United States. Such actions occur in the form of legislation, policy development, research support and supplemental funding. In order to validate and support these actions, there is a need to demonstrate that education is result-ing in increased skills for U.S. citizens. A set of articulated learning outcome expectations can provide definition to quality of life and information about expected outcomes can lead to better decision making.

Exit outcomes are derived from real life role functions (Spady, 1994). Communities that have gone through a consensus building process to determine such outcomes arrive at a set of statements that clearly articulate their expectations of those aspects associated with the requirements found in real-life situations (Spady, 1992b). As more and more communities (local and state-wide) participate in such a process, it becomes evident that there is a set of common expectations. The common set of exit outcome expectations can serve as targets for national expectations (or standards).

Given a set of exit outcomes that help to establish national stan-dards, learner data around these outcomes can serve to assist those at the national level to make more appropriate decisions. At this level, learning outcome data are particularly pertinent to decisions concerning instructional or program research efforts and to identifying program areas in need of supplemental funding. Naturally, if legislators are to appropriate dollars for program improvement, they also will want some learning outcome data to ensure accountability.

The national effort on learning outcomes is indirect and represents only part of what is being done. A large percentage of the national effort is intended to more directly influence and change the system. Policies and regulations are directed toward changing system behavior first. Therefore, national representatives need outcome data that describe changes in the system. For example, policies related to least restrictive environment (LRE) are intended to ensure more opportunities for students with disabilities to become full participants in the community. Those at the national level will be interested in data that show evidence of students participating in general school environments as well as data that show that these students are participants in communities after leaving school (i.e., both system and actualized outcomes).

Another example is evident in policies related to transition from school. These policies are intended to influence the ability of students with disabilities to find and maintain employment and community living opportunities after leaving school. Data that describe employment and community living conditions of students who leave school are critical to determining the extent to which transition policies are achieving the intended effects. Likewise, such data can be used to influence and support the development of future policy, as has happened with the transition from school policies.

Part of the national role is to secure federal dollars that provide direct support to students (e.g., purchase of supplemental services). Decisions and accountability assurances are best monitored through the use of learning outcome data, most specifically exit outcome data. However, a larger national effort is concerned with whether education (as a system) is on track and is affecting the quality of life throughout the nation (i.e., whether lives are enhanced by education). These needs are more specifically addressed through the use of both actualized and system outcome data.

State level. At the state level, the scope of responsibility focuses on each local entity (e.g., each school or each district). State level actions and decisions must support the local entity's efforts to produce quality learners. Even though the state does not provide direct day to day instruction, the constitutional authority and responsibility for public education rests with the state. Therefore, state education agency (SEA) employees are heavily vested in learning outcomes, both exit and enabling.

Learning outcome data can assist state level staff in identifying those program improvement areas that require support. Additionally, learning outcome data can assist state staff in ascertaining the extent to which common expectations for students across the state are being met. Because students most likely will not live in one community all of their lives, and because states must be concerned with maintaining a state-wide quality of life, state representatives will want to identify outcomes that are pertinent to all at the local level. Determining the extent to which students generally are demonstrating behaviors associated with these outcomes is critical to the need to assess the state as a whole. In such an assessment, data can be used to determine the level of supports or program improvement efforts that are needed for each local entity.

A second need for learning outcome data is for analyzing policy decisions that guide and support program improvement and implementation at the local level. A third use is for communicating with legislators to assure that legislative decisions promote student learning and that fiscal resources are invested wisely. Finally, a fourth use of learning outcome data at the state level is to produce a state-wide picture that describes demonstrated learning throughout the state.

Those working at the state level do not have the luxury of having immediate, day to day interaction with students and communities. They also do not make decisions about individual students, but make generalizations about students. Therefore, relying on learning outcomes alone would result in making decisions with only partial information.

Post-school outcome data take on a prominent role. Such data assist SEA personnel in continually checking the relevance and appropriateness of state and district outcome expectations. They also help to identify those areas where the education system interfaces with the larger social system. This helps to identify supports or interventions needed from other agencies that are part of the larger system. Finally, they are critical to assuring the public that education is related to quality of life after school, rather than merely a set of isolated steps one must tolerate and through which one must move.

Additionally, a major function of the state is one of support to education through policy making and resource distribution. Policies and resources generally do not affect the learner directly; rather, they affect the system that supports the learner and reflect the valued expectations that the system is to meet. Therefore, data about the system are critical to good policy decisions. School exit rates (e.g., graduation and dropout rates), opportunities for participation, available community supports, teacher demonstrated skill and available resources are examples of system outcomes we expect. As stated earlier, they do not guarantee acquisition of learning outcomes by students, but they do reflect valued expectations that are critical for sustaining learning outcomes.

For state systems to be outcome-based, such systems will need an equal amount of learning, actualized and system outcome data. Clearly, learning outcomes form the basis of the original OBE movement. Adding actualized and system outcomes broadens the scope and potential use for outcome based decision making about education at the state level.

Local level. At the local level, the scope and specificity is narrower, and the greatest amount of attention is devoted to learning outcomes. Parents need to be assured that the educational content deemed important for their children is that which will lead to acquisition of skills and knowledge critical to real life roles. The community needs assurance that schooling will lead to qualified employees and skilled community members. All community members need data that illustrate that their children are learning and demonstrating skills that will lead to productive and active participation in the community.

Administrators at the local level also need learning outcome data, both exit and enabling, in order to provide the appropriate resources in accordance with student learning needs. Resources include human, technological and fiscal allocations.

Follow-up data that show students working and functioning independently in a community can help verify that the skills taught and learned in school are consistent with the skills needed for jobs and other adult duties in the community. Therefore, information associated with actualized outcomes (e.g., post-school success) cannot be ignored at the local level. Such data are critical to assessing the appropriateness of the articulated learning outcomes to real life expectations. Additionally, system data (e.g., attendance or graduation rates, resource availability by school) are valuable for identifying problems that have an impact on student learning. Low attendance or high dropout rates signify problems and are needed to direct local educator efforts for improving school environments or learning conditions. Many students and families require supports from the community service system in order to fully participate as contributing community members. Both system and actualized outcome data (e.g., healthy life styles or employment characteristics) are critical for working with the larger community to assess community supports that are available and to identify additional supports that will be needed to assure that students can actualize the expected learning outcomes.

Classroom level. Ultimately, and perhaps most importantly, the OBE process focuses on what to teach and how to teach it at the classroom level. Teachers almost exclusively attend to learning outcomes. Learning expectations, both exit and enabling outcomes, are used to develop instructional plans. The immediate concern of a teacher is to have clearly identified annual expectations (i.e., the expected exit outcomes to be achieved by the end of the year) from which short-term unit outcomes can be derived. However, it also is important to know and understand the ultimate exit outcome (i.e., that which the student is expected to know and do upon exiting school) as well as the expectation at the next level (i.e., elementary to middle to high school) in order to assure that the identified annual and subsequent unit outcomes are connected and will lead to the desired, ultimate exit outcome. When we know that students are expected to demonstrate the skills necessary for living on their own when they leave high school, we can determine what that means for skill development at each grade along the way and assure that our instruction is tied to real-life relevant expectations.

With the inclusion of transition as a required component of secondary IEPs, secondary teachers are expected to connect in-school instruction to post-school expectations or desired results. With the passage of the School To Work Opportunities Act of 1994, more attention is being given throughout all of the secondary level to that which students are expected to do when they leave school. This focus is expected in turn to influence the skills that students are taught while in school.

CONCLUSION

Outcome-based education is not a quick fix or product to apply. Rather, it is a new way of thinking and making decisions about education. It is a process that requires determining the desired end result and making certain that all actions and decisions support achieving that desired result.

Even though outcome in its simplest form is equated with result, identifying a common set of outcomes has not proven to be an easy task, partially because individuals have different ideas about outcome depending on how they are applying the term. Applying various types of outcomes to various situations based on decisions to be made can help diminish some of the confusion. Learning, actualized and system outcomes have been proposed as three types of outcomes that are generally identified as relevant to improving education for students with disabilities.

While OBE in its origin was applied primarily at the classroom or instructional level, it can be applied to the entire education system. If there is allowance for different uses for the term "outcomes," e.g., learning, actualized and system outcomes, and if there is willingness to define, clarify and match the type of outcome with the needs of the different components of the system, the principles that started with the OBE movement and the data collected from an outcome-driven perspective can be used effectively throughout the entire system.

REFERENCES

Brolin, D.E. (1989). *Life-centered career education: A competency based approach* (3rd ed.). Reston, VA: The Council for Exceptional Children.

Capitol Publications Inc. (1993). Congress will reconsider national school delivery standards. *Report on Education Research,* January 20.

Chadsey-Rusch, J., Rusch, F.R., & O'Reilly, M.F. (1991). Transition from school to integrated communities. *Remedial and Special Education,* 12(6), 23-33.

Cohen, S.A., & Hyman, I.S. (1993). From Carroll to Bloom: The origin of a great idea. *Outcomes,* 12(3), 5-9.

Darling-Hammond, L. (July, 1992). *Standards of practice for learner-centered schools.* New York, New York: National Center for Restructuring Education, Schools, and Teaching, Teachers College, Columbia University.

DeStefano, L., & Wagner, M. (1990). *Outcome assessment in special education: Lessons learned.* Menlo Park, CA: Transition Institute at Illinois, University of Illinois at Urbana-Champaign, and SRI International.

Frey, W.D., Lynch, L., & Jakwerth, P. (1991). *Educational outcomes for students with disabilities.* East Lansing, MI: Disability Research System, Inc.

Glatthorn, A.A. (1993). Outcome-based education: Reform and the curriculum process. *Journal of Curriculum and Supervision,* 8(4), 354-363.

National Governors' Association (NGA) (1993). Strategic investment: Tough choices for America's future. *Backgrounder,* January 31.

O'Neil, J. (1993). Making sense of outcome-based education. *Instructor,* January, 46-47.

Shavelson, R., McDonnell, L., & Oakes, J. (1989). *Indicators for monitoring mathematics and science education.* Santa Monica, CA: RAND Corporation.

Spady, W.G. (1992a). It's time to take a close look at outcome-based education. *Communique,* 20(6), 16-18.

Spady, W.G. (1992b). Conference handouts. Implementing Transformational Outcome-Based Education, February 7-9; San Antonio, Texas. Conference sponsored by The Center for Peak Performing Schools, Denver, CO.

Spady, W.G. (1994). Choosing outcomes of significance. *Educational Leadership,* 51(6), 18-22.

Wagner, M., Newman, L., D'Amico, R., Jay, E.D., Butler-Nalin, P., Marder, C., & Cox, R. (1991). *Youth with disabilities: How are they doing? The first comprehensive sport from the National Longitudinal Transition Study of Special Education Students.* Menlo Park, CA: SRI International.

Ysseldyke, J.E., Thurlow, M.L., Bruininks, R.H., Gilman, C.J., Deno, S.L., McGrew, K.S., & Shriner, J. G. (1992c). *An evolving conceptual model of educational outcomes for children and youth with disabilities* (Working Paper 2). Minneapolis, MN: National Center on Educational Outcomes.

A State Level Approach to Gathering Data

LaMonte Wyche, Sr.

Howard University

Bob Algozzine

University of North Carolina-Charlotte

Michael L. Vanderwood

University of Minnesota

SUMMARY. What are the ways in which a model of outcomes and indicators can be used by state agencies? Many states are in the process of identifying educational outcomes, but have not yet thought about how to collect data. In this article, we review three applications of a model of outcomes to the collection of data. One application is examining the extent to which students are benefiting from their educational experiences, another the extent to which they are achieving IEP objectives, and another the development of transition IEPs.

To what extent is education working in America? If you were asked to address that question, how would you know? What kinds of data would you gather? Suppose the Chair of the Board of Education in your school district asked you to demonstrate that education was working in the district. Or, more specifically, that

---

Address correspondence to: Bob Algozzine, University of North Carolina-Charlotte, 3135 Colvard, Charlotte, NC 28223.

[Haworth co-indexing entry note]: "A State Level Approach to Gathering Data." Wyche, LaMonte, Sr., Bob Algozzine, and Michael L. Vanderwood. Co-published simultaneously in *Special Services in the Schools* (The Haworth Press, Inc.) Vol. 9, No. 2, 1994, pp. 93-98; and: *Educational Outcomes for Students with Disabilities* (ed: James E. Ysseldyke, and Martha L. Thurlow) The Haworth Press, Inc., 1994, pp. 93-98. Multiple copies of this article/chapter may be purchased from The Haworth Document Delivery Center [1-800-3-HAWORTH; 9:00 a.m. - 5:00 p.m. (EST)].

education was working for students with disabilities. What data would you provide?

The common response to demonstrating that education works for students with disabilities has been to provide child count data. Such data are sensitive to input and process (such as numbers or kinds of students served) but do not reflect outcome. The National Center on Educational Outcomes (NCEO) convened a meeting in September 1993 for the purpose of identifying new ways of demonstrating accountability for special education. The results of that meeting were summarized in an article by Ysseldyke, Thurlow, and Geenen (1993). They identified the following as alternative ways to demonstrate accountability:

1. *Focus on Results or Outcomes.* This involves SEA or LEA specification of desired criteria that must be achieved by students through outcomes-based assessments, and measurement of the extent to which the criteria are achieved.
2. *Collect IEP Information.* This involves tracking the progress of individual students toward accomplishment of IEP objectives, and the aggregation of data on student progress.
3. *Conduct Secondary Analyses on Extant Data.* This requires obtaining existing databases, sorting out students with disabilities, and analyzing data on the performance of those students.
4. *Give Norm-Referenced Tests.* This involves administration at periodic intervals (e.g., grades 4, 8 and 12) of norm-referenced achievement tests to students with disabilities, and reports on the performance of the students.
5. *Create Accreditation Programs.* This requires SEAs to develop criteria for effective delivery of services to students with disabilities, and monitoring of the extent to which LEAs meet those criteria. LEAs that meet criteria are then accredited.

This article addresses the first two points, and illustrates ways in which states are performing these activities. These state examples provide evidence of some of the ways that the NCEO conceptual model can be used to help meet the day-to-day needs of SEA personnel. (Additional examples of applying the NCEO model may be found in Lange and Ysseldyke, this volume.)

USING A CONCEPTUAL MODEL
OF OUTCOMES AND INDICATORS

The National Center on Educational Outcomes developed a conceptual model on educational outcomes and indicators for students with disabilities (Ysseldyke & Thurlow, this volume). The model was developed to provide a framework from which states, districts and schools could develop their own outcomes and indicators. The issue of relevance in this article is the extent to which states use the model to gather data on outcomes. Three states have used the NCEO model for this purpose.

In January 1994 personnel in the District of Columbia (DC) Public Schools started an 18-month project. Working in collaboration with the faculty in the Department of Human Development Psychoeducational Studies at Howard University and NCEO personnel, the DC State Office of Special Education began examining the feasibility of using the NCEO model of educational outcomes and indicators to develop outcome accountability measures for students with disabilities. Project staff are examining (a) the kinds of problems educators encounter when they evaluate the effectiveness of special education, (b) the most appropriate evaluation designs to use, (c) the instruments and methodologies that are most appropriate for evaluating the effectiveness of special education, and (d) the kinds of data analysis procedures that are appropriate for evaluating program effectiveness. The NCEO *Self-Study Guide to the Development of Educational Outcomes and Indicators* (Ysseldyke & Thurlow, 1993) is being used to guide project leaders through the step-by-step process of developing outcomes and indicators. The *Self-Study Guide* is discussed by Thurlow, Ysseldyke, Vanderwood, and Spande, this volume.

First, project leaders established an Advisory Council to direct project efforts. The Council is comprised of special education administrators and teachers from the District, parents, a representative from the DC City Council, a representative of the Center for Minority Research in Special Education, and a representative of NCEO. At its first meeting, the Council decided to accept the NCEO definitions of terms like outcomes and indicators, the NCEO assumptions for development of a conceptual model, and the overall NCEO model as a starting point for the evaluation of special education in the DC Public Schools. Project members formed three groups of stakeholders to participate in Multiattribute Consensus Building (see Vanderwood & Erickson, this volume) in order to refine the model, outcomes and indicators. The mixed groups were comprised of educators, parents, and members of the community. The groups adapted the overall model to their own purposes, and made minor modifications in the wording of some of the indicators.

Using the indicators developed by the three groups of stakeholders, project personnel developed a survey to be filled out by teachers for each student in their program. The survey was completed during summer, 1994 on students who were in 12th grade during the 1993-94 academic year. Data are being aggregated and will be included in a report on pupil performance.

Project personnel in the DC schools were able to apply the NCEO conceptual model of outcomes and indicators to their own local situation, and use the model with minimal modifications.

OUTCOMES APPROACH TO TRANSITION PLANNING

Personnel in the New Jersey Department of Education are using an outcomes approach to move the accountability focus of special education beyond access and procedural compliance. The goal is to improve individual performances in ways that will lead to their having more independent adult lives as productive members in the community. Osowski (1993) outlined several benefits of using an outcomes approach, and identified ways in which the model might be applied to this effort.

First, when an outcomes approach is used, special education is focused on what pupils with disabilities *can do* rather than on what they cannot do. Educators become more concerned with the abilities of pupils than with their disabilities or deficiencies. School personnel develop special education delivery systems through which all decisions about pupils are based on specific educational needs rather than on a disability label or category.

The second advantage of using an outcomes accountability approach is that it is possible to give substance to the elusive transition area between school and adult life. Educators and parents now are required to collaborate in developing and implementing transition plans that are focused on appropriate post-secondary outcomes in the areas of employment, further education, community living, and recreation. The focus is shifted from one of school completion (graduation, completion of course units) to preparation for adult life. State personnel can use the NCEO models of outcomes and indicators at school completion and post-school levels, translating specific indicators into objectives for transition IEPs.

A third advantage to using an outcomes accountability approach is that it provides an opportunity to give meaning to the placement of pupils with disabilities in regular education classes with supportive services and accommodations. When transition IEPs include clear objectives indicating the outcomes students are to achieve, expectations for pupil performance are clearly defined, and the extent to which additional special services are needed is clearer.

The fourth advantage of using an outcomes accountability approach to develop transition IEPs is that it gives the SEA an opportunity to monitor program improvement (as opposed to identifying districts that are noncompliant with procedural requirements). LEA personnel, in turn, are able to direct their energies toward helping students achieve IEP objectives and to spend less time working toward procedural compliance.

A fifth advantage identified by Osowski is that educators are able to have data on the effectiveness of their educational strategies and programs. As in the DC Public Schools, specifying student outcomes and collecting data on student achievement of those outcomes provides SEA personnel evidence of program effectiveness.

AGGREGATION OF DATA ON IEP ACCOMPLISHMENTS

Five Area Education Agencies (AEAs) in Iowa are using curriculum-based measurement procedures to monitor pupil progress toward the accomplishment of IEP objectives. Graphing procedures are used to provide information that teachers, in turn, use to make instructional changes. The approach is not unlike that used in many states and LEAs across the U.S. What is unique is the way in which the information is aggregated.

SEA and AEA personnel in Iowa have been identifying "standard tasks," performance measures that can be used across schools or districts to describe student progress. Standard tasks have been identified for some academic areas, and groups of school personnel are busy identifying tasks in the areas of preschool education, social skills, secondary and transitional education, and health. It is the intent of the project ultimately to link these measures of outcomes and domains to the NCEO model. It is thought that it will be possible to aggregate data on IEP accomplishments (performance on standard tasks), and to use this information as evidence of outcomes accomplishments.

The Iowa Department of Education recently brought together teachers and administrators from participating AEAs to analyze and give feedback to hypothetical results collected using domains from the NCEO model. Results of that working session indicated positive support for the idea of IEP aggregation, with participants viewing such information as valuable in crafting staff development initiatives and teacher self-evaluation.

CONCLUSION

A conceptual model of outcomes and indicators can be applied by states to enhance the extent to which individuals with disabilities profit from their educational programs. The examples included in this article illustrate three applications of an outcomes accountability approach. Other articles in this volume illustrate ways in which states can develop their own systems of outcomes and indicators, and match the NCEO model to their own goals or standards.

REFERENCES

Osowski, J. (1993). Outcomes move educational focus beyond access and procedural compliance. *Outcomes, 3.*

Ysseldyke, J. E., & Thurlow, M. L. (1993). *Self-study guide to the development of educational outcomes and indicators.* Minneapolis, MN: National Center on Educational Outcomes.

Ysseldyke, J. E., Thurlow, M. L., & Geenen, K. (1993). *Implementation of alternative methods for making educational accountability decisions for students with disabilities* (Synthesis Report 12). Minneapolis, MN: National Center on Educational Outcomes.

Consensus Building

Michael L. Vanderwood
Ron Erickson

University of Minnesota

SUMMARY. The National Center on Educational Outcomes (NCEO) has used a Multi-Attribute Consensus Building (MACB) technique to build consensus on a national model of educational outcomes and indicators. MACB is a computer-based process that facilitates group decision making for a variety of purposes. It requires development of a list and selecting specific items from the list. MACB uses group and individual ratings of indicators to help stakeholders come to agreement on indicators of educational outcomes that should be selected. NCEO used MACB to establish educational indicators and outcomes, thereby creating a model of outcomes. The stages of consensus building and tasks that must be accomplished in each stage are described in detail.

With pressure to restructure the educational system at state and local levels, many different groups are involved in suggesting changes and how to make them happen. This is true as we attempt

The preparation of this manuscript was supported in part by a Cooperative Agreement (H159C00004) between the U.S. Department of Education, Office of Special Education Programs and the University of Minnesota. Points of view or opinions do not necessarily reflect those of the Department of Education or offices within it.

Address correspondence to: Michael L. Vanderwood, 350 Elliott Hall, 75 East River Road, University of Minnesota, Minneapolis, MN 55455.

[Haworth co-indexing entry note]: "Consensus Building." Vanderwood, Michael L., and Ron Erickson. Co-published simultaneously in *Special Services in the Schools* (The Haworth Press, Inc.) Vol. 9, No. 2, 1994, pp. 99-113; and: *Educational Outcomes for Students with Disabilities* (ed: James E. Ysseldyke, and Martha L. Thurlow) The Haworth Press, Inc., 1994, pp. 99-113. Multiple copies of this article/chapter may be purchased from The Haworth Document Delivery Center [1-800-3-HAWORTH; 9:00 a.m. - 5:00 p.m. (EST)].

99

to develop a meaningful system for assessing the condition of education. Building consensus among various groups of stakeholders is critical to ensuring full participation (Blank, 1993). In its effort to develop a system of educational outcomes and indicators, the National Center on Educational Outcomes (NCEO) chose to use a process that would build consensus among educators, policymakers, administrators, parents, and other stakeholders (Ysseldyke, Thurlow, Bruininks, Oilman, Deno, McGrew, & Shriner, 1992).

To identify the process it would use, NCEO reviewed several different approaches. The decision was made to modify an evaluation system used in the management sciences. Multiattribute Utility Evaluation (MAU) is an evaluation model that is designed to facilitate decision making about several different options or alternatives (see Lewis, Erickson, Johnson, and Bruininks, 1991, for a detailed description of MAU).

MACB is a quantitative, objective approach for determining a small group's opinion about the importance of each item in a list. Specifically, consensus is created by requiring each member of a group to rate the importance of each item on a list (no matter how many items) from 0 to 100, presenting to the group each member's ratings and averages for each item, and then facilitating discussion around items that have a relatively large range of ratings. Computer technology is used to record ratings and calculate descriptive statistical information about the ratings. It is also used to facilitate the display and modification of items that may be made prior to the rating of the items. With this approach, discussion is focused on presenting and understanding various viewpoints regarding specific items about which members disagree. After hearing different viewpoints, members are allowed to change their ratings, giving an objective indication of the extent to which the group agrees on the importance of each item. The computer technology enables participants to view the effects of changed ratings immediately upon changing ratings.

NCEO used the MACB process to help generate and reach agreement on the outcomes and indicators that are included in a model of educational outcomes (see article by Ysseldyke and Thurlow in this volume for a representation of the model). NCEO produced, with input from many individuals, large lists of outcomes and indicators and used MACB to determine how important these indicators were to various groups. MACB conferences were held with several groups of parents, educators, and administrators (for a more detailed description of the use of MACB at NCEO see Ysseldyke and Thurlow, 1993). After gaining input from these groups, NCEO used their ratings to determine which indicators and outcomes to use in the model.

DESCRIPTION OF THE PROCESS

When using the MACB approach to identify outcomes and indicators (as NCEO did), three general stages are involved: Generation of Input, Consensus Conference, and Synthesis of Consensus. Figure 1 portrays the three stages of the process and the tasks that must be accomplished during each stage.

Before beginning the process, a conceptual model that includes a basic framework of outcomes and the purpose of the consensus building process must be delineated. The initial framework that we used at NCEO to begin the process was that presented in "What Results . . . " by Ysseldyke and Thurlow in this volume, and our goal was both to obtain input on our model and to have the participants develop and come to consensus on a list of indicators of the outcomes.

Stage I: Generation of input. The first MACB stage is indicator generation. To accomplish this task, participants representing stakeholder groups must be identified and at least 4 but not more than 10 individuals must be selected. Group processing is easier to facilitate and occurs more rapidly with groups of 10 or fewer. Depending upon the purpose of the meeting, the group can be a mixture of several different types of stakeholders (e.g., parents, teachers, administrators) or it can be comprised of members from just one stakeholder group.

After the participants are identified, they are sent the current conceptual model. They are asked to review the model, generate a specific number of indicators for each domain in the model, and return the list. NCEO requested that each participant generate four indicators for each outcome domain and return the list approximately one week before the MACB conference.

FIGURE 1. Multi-Attribute Consensus Building: Stages and Tasks to Accomplish

Before the Process Begins

♦ Develop conceptual model

♦ Determine stakeholder groups–These should be groups influenced by the finished product.

Stage I
Generation of Input

1. Select 4 to 10 stakeholders to attend the working session.

2. Have stakeholders generate indicators for each outcome domain.

3. Develop a master list of indicators for each outcome area.

4. Create a spreadsheet shell that computes the average and range of the ratings for each indicator.

5. Prepare for stakeholder working session (e.g., make copies of ratings sheets, etc.).

Stage II
Consensus Working Session

Introduction
1. Explain purpose of meeting.
2. Describe MACB process.
3. Tell participants how information will be used.

Clarification
1. Present master list of indicators for one outcome domain.
2. Allow participants to make modifications to indicators if group agrees. Computer operator modifies master list.
3. Limit discussion to wording and meaning of indicators.

Rating
1. Participants rate the importance of each indicator (0 - 100).
2. One indicator must be 100.
3. Computer operator enters information into spreadsheet.

Discussion
1. Review average ratings for each indicator with stakeholders.
2. Discuss indicators with large ranges in ratings or mid-range average ratings (60 - 80).
3. Encourage revisions to ratings after discussion.

Stage III
Synthesis of Consensus

1. Compute standard deviation, median, and number of individuals who rated each indicator greater than 75 and less than 50.

2. Identify indicators with very high and very low average ratings. Keep those with very high ratings.

3. Make decisions about remaining unclear items. Use other indices and staff judgment to clarify the importance of the indicator.

After all lists have been returned, a master list for each area must be developed that includes the respondents' lists as well as indicators developed by the staff or previous groups. All indicators should be phrased in a similar format; no duplicate indicators should appear. A sample of indicators developed during this stage is presented in Table 1.

Stage II: Consensus conference. The MACB conference is the second stage of the process. It is the stage in which consensus building occurs. It is desirable to have at least two staff members to run the meeting, which can last from half a day to two or three days. The length of the conference is determined by the number of outcomes and indicators that need to be rated and the number of individuals who attend. One staff member serves as the facilitator/moderator while the other operates the computer. Both members should be familiar with the outcomes and indicators, and issues that may arise during discussion about them.

Presenting a detailed explanation of the process and the purpose of the meeting before beginning is essential. It is also important to mention how the information gathered from the participants will be used. After this, the facilitator introduces the first outcome domain and starts the consensus building activity. Consensus building consists of three parts: clarification, rating, and discussion.

During *clarification,* the facilitator presents the list of indicators to the groups and asks for questions about the wording. Group members are allowed to modify the statements if the rest of the

TABLE 1. Initial List of Indicators for School Completion for Physical Health

A. Percent of students who indicate that they use tobacco products
B. Percent of students who make good nutritional choices
C. Percent of students who have abused alcohol or drugs in the past year
D. Percent of students who indicate they have had unprotected sex in the past year
E. Percent of students who elect to participate in sports, recreational, and/or exercise activities
F. Percent of students who are aware of basic safety precautions and procedures
G. Percent of students who are aware of basic fitness needs
H. Percent of students who are aware of basic health care needs
 I. Percent of students who know when, where, and how to access health care
J. Percent of students who are physically fit

group agrees. The computer operator makes changes on the computer, which is connected to an overhead projection display that allows the group members to see each change that is made. This time should only be spent to clarify the indicators and add any that are considered necessary by the group. An effort must be made by the facilitator during this period to prevent the group from focusing too much time on the wording of an indicator. Clarification is the purpose here, not extensive wordsmithing.

After the clarification step, the facilitator starts the *rating* process by requesting participants to write down each indicator on a rating sheet and rate each one from 0 to 100 based on its importance, where 100 represents a very important indicator. The only requirement is that at least one indicator must be considered the most important and rated a 100. Other indicators that are considered to be equally important may also be rated 100.

As each participant completes the rating sheet, it is given to the computer operator, who enters the ratings into a spreadsheet on the computer. The spreadsheet is designed to display each member's ratings and the group's range and average for each indicator (see example display in Figure 2). This format can be created on most spreadsheet software (e.g., MicroSoft Excel™, LOTUS 123™). As the ratings are entered into the computer, the operator checks to make sure that each participant has rated at least one indicator 100 and that all members rate all indicators. By giving the rating sheets to the computer operator as they are completed by individuals, the data entry process can be finished almost immediately after the last sheet is received.

After all ratings are entered into the computer, the entire group's ratings are reviewed on the overhead projector. From these, the facilitator helps to create group *discussion* about those indicators that have a large range and high degree of variability among ratings. Individuals who have given ratings on a specific indicator that are at the low or high end of the ratings are asked to present their opinions about the indicator. This is done especially with those individuals who have ratings that could be considered outliers. If it appears that all members are in agreement about a specific indicator, discussion is not required on that indicator.

Throughout the discussion process, the facilitator encourages

FIGURE 2. Example of Stakeholder Ratings Display

	NV	PD	DF	MD	LH	DC	AM	CV	AVG	MIN	MAX
A	90	50	80	80	70	50	80	60	70	50	90
B	95	90	70	100	90	90	80	75	86	70	100
C	90	30	10	60	90	40	60	80	58	10	90
D	80	30	50	80	80	50	80	70	65	30	80
E	100	100	100	90	100	100	100	100	99	90	100
F	95	100	80	100	100	95	90	65	91	65	100

participants to feel free to change their ratings after they have heard other opinions. The discussion step is the most important part of the process, and the part that helps bring the group to consensus. Therefore, the facilitator must ensure that discussion is focused on indicators where differences in ratings exist. After the discussion of all indicators with discrepancies is finished, the facilitator moves on to the next domain and begins the clarification process. This three part procedure continues until consensus is reached for all desired domains.

Stage III: Synthesis of consensus. The final stage of MACB is completed after the conference. The selection process is generally based on the data, but for borderline cases, the decision should be based upon statements made during the rating process and other factors concerning the indicator (such as feasibility of use or similarity to other indicators already chosen). Several different indices of central tendency and variation can easily be produced using spreadsheet formulas. Along with the standard deviation, median, range, and mean, we used the number of individuals who rated an indicator higher than 75 and the number with ratings lower than 50 as useful indices of a group's consensus on a specific indicator. The breakoff points were arbitrarily selected based on experience with ratings.

Although complex combinations of statistical criteria could be used to direct decision making (Lewis et al., 1991), NCEO experiences from nearly 10 different conferences suggest that a simple approach is quite adequate for making good decisions. The first cut of the indicators is achieved by looking at the average ratings. The general rule is to keep ones with high average ratings above 90 and drop those with low average ratings below 50.

TECHNICAL AND LOGISTICAL ISSUES

One of the unique features of MACB is the use of a computer, spreadsheet and word processing software, overhead projector, and a computer display projection panel to expedite the consensus building process and provide feedback to the stakeholder group. Several different combinations of equipment are known to work. When determining which type of computer to use, several factors must be considered. First, the computer must be able to connect to a display panel that allows the computer screen to be displayed on a projection screen through an overhead projector. Second, meeting facilitators and computer operators need to be familiar with the chosen software and the computer. The MACB conference computer operator needs to know how to solve problems that might arise, and be very adept at entering, changing and saving text and data. The speed of the computer is the third factor that must be considered. Although a fast computer is not essential, the process can become painstakingly slow if it takes an extraordinary amount of time to enter data and update the display.

TECHNICAL CHARACTERISTICS
OF THE MACB PROCESS

Webster defines *consensus* as "group solidarity in sentiment and belief." But how much solidarity should one expect through the use of the MACB process? Some of the questions that arise about the technical characteristics of MACB were answered in a recent use of the process. Stakeholders in an urban Minnesota school district used the MACB method to assist in an evaluation of their educational services to secondary students with learning disabilities. The administrative sponsors of the evaluation constructed a two-tiered model of effectiveness, consisting of educational domains and accompanying effectiveness indicators within each domain. The assembled stakeholder group was asked to assign importance ratings, first to the four major domains, and then to each of the four groups of effectiveness indicators.

To investigate the presence of consensus, comparatively low standard deviations were interpreted to reflect higher levels of consensus among the ratings of individual stakeholders. In 14 out of 16 cases (87.5%), the standard deviations of ratings were less than 20 points of importance. Only in two cases was the standard deviation of ratings larger. Results also suggested that consensus may have improved during the process; standard deviations averaged 16.67 during the initial rating of domains, but fell to an average of 5.93 during the final round of ratings.

The question of reliability with a technique such as MACB is focused primarily on the technique's ability to produce similar results with different groups. One way to measure this is to start with the same set of indicators with two or more groups and examine the difference in average ratings for each indicator across groups. The wording of the indicators must also be examined to determine whether a group changed the meaning of an indicator while rewording it.

OTHER USES OF THE MACB PROCESS

MACB is well suited for any type of group decision making that requires development of a list and then selecting specific items from the list. Although NCEO has only used this process in helping select educational outcomes and indicators, MACB has been used by others to help define and select research priorities, to help identity educational outcomes of university graduate level training programs, and to facilitate strategic planning by identifying critical educational issues in the next 20 years.

OTHER DECISION SUPPORT STRATEGIES

As a method that serves to facilitate better decision-making, multiattribute consensus building shares some common characteristics with other decision support strategies. Two well-accepted and well-researched methods of consensus building are the Delphi survey technique and the Nominal Group Technique. While these strategies share common characteristics with the MACB method, there are notable differences in their comparative reliance on stakeholders, and in the types of problems for which they were designed.

The Delphi survey technique. In ancient Greek history, Delphi was the site of the oracle of Apollo, a place where high priests would forecast the future by interpreting the entrails of sacrificed animals. The approach bears this namesake because its developers Dalkey (1967) and Helmer (1967) designed it as a means by which future trends could be more accurately predicted and anticipated within a corporate setting. Working as physicist and futurist for Rand Corporation, they applied Delphi to help solve crucial U.S. Department of Defense contract problems.

Many researchers have since used the Delphi method and expanded its application beyond its original focus on prediction. In actual use the procedures are easily modified to meet the situational context and the nature of the task. Its developers suggest that it can be effective for the following purposes: (a) to determine and develop a range of possible program alternatives; (b) to seek out information that may generate a consensus on the part of the respondent group; (c) to explore or expose underlying assumptions or information leading to different judgments; (d) to correlate informed judgments on a topic spanning a wide range of disciplines, or (e) to educate the respondent group about the diverse and interrelated aspects of the topic. In brief, a Delphi survey technique is used to collect perceptions or opinions from stakeholders on a predetermined set of ideas laid out by expert opinion.

The Nominal Group Technique. Delp, Thesen, Motiwalla, and Seshadri (1977) define Nominal Group Technique (NGT) as "a group process for eliciting opinions and aggregating judgments to increase rationality and creativity when faced with an unstructured problem situation." Its title stems from the method's characteristic of requiring members of a group to work in each other's presence, but with nominal interaction. Credit for its original development is generally given to Delbecq, Van de Ven, and Gustafson (1975).

At the beginning of an NGT meeting, a question is posed to a group made up of no more than 10 individuals. The question may seek ideas about the criteria by which to judge a program, the present needs within an organization, or the key components of an agency mission statement–the process is adaptable to many situations. Each member then independently and silently lists his or her responses to the question. Following a reasonable amount of time, the group leader asks each member in round-robin fashion to report a *single* answer while the leader writes it down for the group to see. While no discussion is allowed during these contributed comments, group members are asked to report whether the response being given duplicates any of their own. In such cases, the duplicity is noted by placing a check after the response, and eliminating similar responses from the lists of other members. This activity continues until everyone's list of answers is exhausted.

The second stage of NGT involves the clarification of each of the contributed responses. The group leader must be careful not to allow argument over whether certain items should be included in the list; the next step will determine that. Instead, discussion should only focus on clarifying the meaning of each response, with members allowed to pose questions to the contributor or other supporters of the response.

It is assumed that in most situations, the list of responses generated by the group in an NGT process may be too large for the purpose intended. During the third stage of this technique, group members are asked to identify and rank order a small number of responses (usually 7 ± 2) from the longer list of items. Small response cards are provided for the group members to record their choices. Cards are collected after a reasonable time, shuffled for anonymity, and tallied in front of the group. Discussion ensues over the most highly rated items, with the group leader directing the group's attention to any highly discrepant scores. After a reasonable amount of discussion about the first set of ranks, a second ranking is performed, with the results of this second round considered final.

Comparisons among methods. The Delphi method, Nominal Group Technique, and MACB all offer rational methodologies for decision making by groups of stakeholder constituents. Perhaps the most readily apparent difference among these approaches is their comparative emphasis on open dialogue and interaction among stakeholders. The Delphi intentionally allows *no* face-to-face contact among respondents; such a constraint is believed to allow for more honest reactions to the opinions reported by other colleagues. The Nominal Group Technique opens the door only slightly wider, allowing statements of clarification and questions among stakeholders at certain points in the process, but preserves anonymity during the final ranking exercises. In contrast to the Delphi and NGT's objective of deriving consensus through limited discourse, MACB provides a forum to allow minority opinions to be fully defended and considered.

During an MACB session, the presence of a very high importance rating in the midst of many low scores (or vice versa) precipitates discussion, led by the facilitator, on the rationale for such diverse scoring. The facilitator does not necessarily seek to change the outlying value through questioning the stakeholder who assigned it. Variability is important to uncover since it could indicate the opinion of a particularly well-informed stakeholder. His or her information base may be more pronounced in regard to a particular aspect of educational service delivery, and therefore is operating with a perspective unique to the group. Such privileged information can be shared with the other group members during the pursuant discussion, in order to allow any revisions by other stakeholders based on the new ideas or information. Likewise, it is possible that the stakeholder is misinformed or is misinterpreting the meaning behind a particular item or idea, and in fact needs the information held by others in the group for clarification.

This open elaboration on rating discrepancies is believed to be an essential requirement in reaching the best possible consensus among the group. In those situations where the divergent scores remain unchanged following discussion, the final averaged rating will likely be only slightly affected by the presence of a single outlying score. However, by allowing the inclusion of ideas that only hold minority support in the overall framework, and encouraging open discussion on those items that may hold very different levels of importance among group members, the MACB model encourages a greater sustained level of involvement, satisfaction and contribution from all members of the stakeholder group.

Through their limitations on discussion, the Delphi and NGT strategies prevent the decision-making process from being overrun by dominant or aggressive participants. However, these processes also forego the invaluable rewards of interactive learning and collaborative conclusions. Most stakeholder groups are a divergent lot; in an educational decision-making context, they may represent both the professional and layperson, and both the provider and consumer of services. Providing open, constructive discourse among these constituents through the MACB methodology has proven to be a promising strategy in improving the level of consensus among stakeholders with varying perspectives.

MACB does have several limitations that need to be recognized by those planning to use the process. First, as with any type of rating system, MACB is susceptible to different response styles of the participants. For example, individuals may use different referent points when rating, always respond in a similar fashion, or only use a certain part of the scale.

Another limitation is that because the indicators are easily modified using the computer, groups often spend a large amount of time attempting to reword the indicators. Modifying an indicator is important if the indicator becomes more clear to the group. However, discussion should generally focus on the ratings and why one person rated an indicator differently from another.

The final limitation of the MACB process is that although everyone has an opportunity to rate and participate in discussion, strong believers can sometimes dominate conversation and prevent others from participating as fully as they desire. One "solution" to this problem that we have used is to always provide participants with a form that they can use to put down their final thoughts, concerns, and reservations about any indicator.

CONCLUSION

For NCEO and its effort to reach consensus about what the important educational outcomes and indicators are, the MACB process has been invaluable. It has made it possible to bring together individuals from very diverse perspectives (e.g., legislators, school administrators, parents, general educators, special educators) and to reach agreement. The process promotes a focus at an objective level, even when the issues being discussed are quite value-laden. And, after completing the process, the participants are sold on the product they have produced, and support the implementation and dissemination of the model.

Developing an accountability system that is based on outcomes will require schools and school systems to solicit ideas from a variety of educational stakeholders, some of whom should represent the perspectives of related services personnel. Special or related services within schools include a variety of professionals who play a critical role in quality educational service delivery. School psychologists, occupational and physical therapists, speech and language specialists, and others can provide unique perspectives on the desired outcomes of our educational efforts and can more effectively design, provide and evaluate their own services when such outcomes are identified in concert with instructional staff, administrators, parents and other interested parties. MACB holds much promise as a means to build this vision of constructive consensus-building.

REFERENCES

Blank, R. K. (1993). Developing a system of education indicators: Selecting, implementing, and reporting indicators. *Educational Evaluation and Policy Analysis, 15*(1), 65-80.

Dalkey, N. C. (1967). *Delphi.* Santa Monica, CA: Rand Corporation.

Delbecq, A., Van de Ven, A., & Gustafson, D. (1975). *Group techniques for program planning: A guide to nominal group and Delphi.* Chicago: Scott Foresman.

Delp, P., Thesen, A., Motiwalla, J., & Seshadri, N. (1977). *Systems tools for project planning.* Bloomington, IN: PASITAM.

Helmer, O. (1967). *Analysis of the future: The delphi method.* Santa Monica, CA: Rand Corporation.

Lewis, D. R., Erickson, R. N., Johnson, D. R., & Bruininks, R. H. (1991). *Using multiattribute utility evaluation techniques in special education.* Unpublished manuscript, University of Minnesota, Institute on Community Integration, Minneapolis.

NCEO. (1993). *State and school district development of educational outcomes and indicators: A guide for self study.* Minneapolis: University of Minnesota, National Center on Educational Outcomes.

Ysseldyke, J. E., & Thurlow, M. L. (1993). *Development of a comprehensive model of educational outcomes and indicators for students with disabilities.* Minneapolis: University of Minnesota, National Center on Educational Outcomes.

Ysseldyke, J. E., Thurlow, M. L., Bruininks, R. H., Oilman, C. J., Deno, S. L., McGrew, K. S., & Shriner, J. G. (1992). *An evolving conceptual model of educational outcomes for children and youth with disabilities.* Minneapolis: University of Minnesota, National Center on Educational Outcomes.

A Guide to Developing and Implementing a System of Outcomes and Indicators

Martha L. Thurlow
James E. Ysseldyke
Michael L. Vanderwood
Gail Spande

National Center on Educational Outcomes
University of Minnesota

SUMMARY. One of the biggest obstacles to focusing on the outcomes of schooling is defining outcomes and coming to agreement on which outcomes to measure. We have worked with stakeholders from throughout the country to develop a national model of outcomes and indicators. In this article, we describe specific steps we have found effective in developing and implementing an outcomes system. We describe how to establish a foundation for such an effort, how to develop a model, considerations in data collection and reporting, and putting an outcomes system in place.

Educators know far more about the kinds of instruction and services students receive, the settings in which they are educated,

---

The preparation of this manuscript was supported in part by a Cooperative Agreement (H159C00004) between the U.S. Department of Education, Office of Special Education Programs and the University of Minnesota. Points of view or opinions do not necessarily reflect those of the Department of Education or offices within it.

Address correspondence to: Martha L. Thurlow, 350 Elliott Hall, 75 East River Road, University of Minnesota, Minneapolis, MN 55455.

[Haworth co-indexing entry note]: "A Guide to Developing and Implementing a System of Outcomes and Indicators." Thurlow, Martha L. et al. Co-published simultaneously in *Special Services in the Schools* (The Haworth Press, Inc.) Vol. 9, No. 2, 1994, pp. 115-126; and: *Educational Outcomes for Students with Disabilities* (ed: James E. Ysseldyke, and Martha L. Thurlow) The Haworth Press, Inc., 1994, pp. 115-126. Multiple copies of this article/chapter may be purchased from The Haworth Document Delivery Center [1-800-3-HAWORTH; 9:00 a.m. - 5:00 p.m. (EST)].

and the resources necessary to educate students than they do about the results they produce. Resources are important: schools everywhere are constantly struggling to maintain quality educational programs in resource-scarce environments. But, the measurement of process should be secondary to the measurement of results (outcomes). Knowledge of educational outcomes is useful because it helps identify the skills and knowledge with which students leave schools, and indicators of these outcomes provide a way to track progress toward achieving the outcomes. Determining how to achieve the results (the process of education) comes after the outcomes are identified.

The purpose of this article is to describe a four step process that we have used at the National Center on Educational Outcomes (NCEO) to develop a national model of educational outcomes and indicators. It was through this process that outcomes and indicators were developed for school completion (Ysseldyke, Thurlow, & Gilman, 1993d), post-school (Ysseldyke, Thurlow, & Gilman, 1993c), and early childhood levels (Ysseldyke, Thurlow, & Gilman, 1993a, 1993b). The NCEO model is an example of a system of outcomes and indicators, and the process we used to develop the model can be used by others.

As states, districts, and schools are called upon to determine the outcomes of education, special services personnel will contribute to the development process. Special services personnel can be leaders in this effort because of their understanding of the diversity of student needs and the need to be accountable for *all* students. The steps that state or local education agency personnel should go through are:

1. Establishment of a solid foundation for assessment efforts,
2. Development, adoption, or adaptation of a model,
3. Establishment of a data collection and reporting system, and
4. Installation of the system.

The full checklist of steps to consider in the development of a system of educational outcomes and indicators is shown in Table 1. Each of the four steps is described in detail below. Examples of implementing the self-study guide may be found in Wyche, Algozzine, and Vanderwood, and Lange and Ysseldyke in this volume.

Although the process of developing a system of educational outcomes and indicators is presented in a linear fashion, the actual development is not nearly that neat. Because the process relies heavily on stakeholder participation, various concerns, issues, and discussions will become apparent that may cause the re-thinking of decisions made earlier. The development of a system of educational outcomes and indicators is an evolutionary process.

TABLE 1. Four Steps in the Development of a System of Educational Outcomes and Indicators

1. Establish a solid foundation for your efforts.

    a. Involve stakeholders up front

    b. Decide why you want to measure outcomes

    c. Define your terms

    d. Consider your assumptions

    e. Resolve the fundamental issues in assessment of outcomes

2. Develop, adopt, or adapt a model.

    a. Select your approach

    b. Define your outcome domains

    c. Define your outcomes

    d. Define your indicators

3. Establish a data collection and reporting system.

    a. Decide where you will get your data

    b. Develop/adapt data collection and analysis mechanisms

    c. Decide how you will report and use the information

4. Install the system.

    a. Create incentives and support for adoption and use

    b. Prepare staff and the public for the changes

    c. Evaluate the system as it is implemented

STEP 1: ESTABLISHING A SOLID FOUNDATION FOR YOUR EFFORTS

Involve stakeholders up front. To successfully implement a system of educational outcomes and indicators, it is necessary to use a planning/advisory group, which includes those who have a stake in implementation of the system. A wide array of participants ensures that important concerns are reflected in the outcomes system. It also provides a way to tap the expertise of others who are knowledgeable about educational issues, the needs of the community, and the realities of school and family life.

State education agency (SEA) or local education agency (LEA) personnel must carefully consider the representation of various groups on a planning committee because the representatives will be the primary communication link to others. General invitations, individual invitations, and nominations for representatives probably will be needed to recruit the participants of the planning advisory group.

The involvement of the stakeholders can take different forms. Some stakeholders may choose to participate as very active members and attend meetings regularly. Others may simply want to be kept informed of progress being made. Still others may be included by way of written communication, fax, or e-mail, but not regularly attend meetings. Some people to consider including in the planning committee are school district personnel, including superintendents, teachers, principals, and representatives from the paraprofessional and clerical staff, parents, students, community members, and representatives from business.

Decide why you want to measure outcomes. There are several uses for outcomes data. First, the information can be used for program improvement. Knowing what programs are working well and which ones need improvement can help determine effective teaching methods and assist in making resource allocation decisions. Second, outcomes data can be used as an accountability tool. The data can be used to determine the extent to which expected educational outcomes are being achieved. Caution should be exercised if this is a primary use of the outcomes data. We believe that negative unintended consequences occur if high stakes are associated with educational programs (such as withholding a diploma, reduction in funding, public display of test scores). Some of the unintended consequences include an increase in the number of students referred to special education, (Allington & McGill-Franzen, 1991), and the possibility of fewer teachers and students willing to take reasonable risks, higher dropout rates, etc. The use of the outcomes system can be a powerful accountability tool, but it should be installed slowly so that it facilitates school improvement, not negative repercussions.

A third use of outcomes data is for public information. The data, aggregated at the school level or higher, can tell the public the extent to which outcomes are achieved. Again, users of the outcomes system are cautioned against publishing data on small groups of students and individual classes for the reasons cited above. Used in a responsible way, public disclosure of the results of schooling, coupled with policies such as school choice, can increase the level of accountability in the school and system. Fourth, the outcomes data can be used for policy formulation. Major decisions, such as how the school is to be organized and how education is to be delivered on a broad scale can be supported with information on the achievement of outcomes combined with process information.

A system of educational outcomes and indicators is a system for collecting data on important aspects of education. Issues such as who will collect the data, who will receive the data, and at which level the data will be reported (individual, class, grade level, school, or district) must be addressed.

A safe place for schools to start may be to aggregate the outcomes information at a grade level or school level, and use the information for program improvement. An example of the use of the information could be to evaluate the effectiveness of involving businesses in the school. If, for example, a desired outcome is student awareness of career options, classes that use businesses for job shadowing and as guest speakers could be compared to classes that teach about job opportunities in a more conventional way. Both the school and the businesses will want to know whether business involvement is an effective use of resources.

Define your terms. Next, with a broad participation base and an understanding of why outcomes are to be measured, key terms need to be defined. Words such as "outcomes" and "indicators" can have several meanings. How these words are defined by NCEO appears in "What Results . . ." by Ysseldyke and Thurlow, this volume. These and other terms, such as "all students," "standards," "outcomes-based education" and "world class," should be defined as they emerge in discussions.

Consider your assumptions. The fourth part of step one is to consider your assumptions. NCEO used a number of assumptions in development of its model of educational outcomes and indicators. Among them were assumptions that: (a) the model would be appropriate for all children, regardless of the characteristics of individuals; (b) the model would primarily focus on intended outcomes, but be sensitive to unintended outcomes as well; (c) the model would reflect the diversity of gender, culture, race and other characteristics of the students in today's school population; and (d) although a comprehensive system of indicators should be based on demonstrated functional relationships between outcome indicators and indicators of educational inputs, contextual characteristics, and processes, valued indicators may be included even if functional relationships have not been established. These are an example of assumptions that will anchor the development of the outcomes and indicators system. Planning advisory committees may wish to use, edit, or add to this list of assumptions.

Resolve fundamental outcomes assessment issues. Key issues include developing one system for all students versus several separate, related systems; whether to differentiate based on age/grade levels; categorical versus non-categorical indicators; whether to differentiate based on ability; system versus individual indicators; and whether to consider enablers and prerequisites as outcomes. It is very important to involve all the stakeholders in these discussions, just as it is in other discussions that form the guiding principles of an outcomes system. After a series of consensus meetings, NCEO decided to develop a system that could be used for all students rather than separate, related systems. NCEO also decided to differentiate based on age/grade levels because of differing expectations across levels. The system was not developed to differentiate between different special education categories, because it was hoped that similar educational outcomes would be attained by all students.

The discussion of system versus individual indicators is an important one. Some parents think that the impact of indicators on their children will be negative because they believe their children cannot reach some outcomes. For example, a student with a severe physical handicap may never meet the outcome of physical fitness. Or a student with severe cognitive impairment may not meet the outcome of reading, writing, and math proficiency. The intent of the NCEO model is that it be used to measure the progress of a system, not as a way to demonstrate that some students have less ability. If the outcomes system is to be used for individuals, it should be done in a realistic and fair way so that students are challenged and adults get information that is useful in designing educational goals for each student.

STEP 2: DEVELOP, ADAPT OR ADOPT A MODEL

Select your approach. The outcomes assessment process should be driven by a conceptual model. A model can be developed for a specific educational system, or a preexisting model can be adopted or adapted. When selecting an approach to use, the assumptions and issues raised in Step 1 must guide the process. With input from several groups of stakeholders, NCEO developed a new model (see Ysseldyke and Thurlow this volume for an example and description of the model). The model contains eight outcome domains and is developmental in nature. This model suggests that resources influence educational opportunity and process, which influences educational outcomes.

Define your outcome domains. Outcome domains define and specify the type of outcomes and indicators that will be developed. In some circumstances, users may only need to focus on academic domains, while others may want to focus on the social or emotional aspects of education. The selection of domains is closely tied to the type of approach used and must also be based on the assumptions and issues raised in Step 1. NCEO's domains are very broad in nature and are designed to give decision makers a complete view of an educational system. The domains of Presence and Participation, and Accommodation and Adaptation, which are normally considered process domains, were included because of stakeholder input.

Many groups thought that these areas are critical for students with disabilities, students with limited English proficiency, and Chapter 1 students.

Define your outcomes and indicators. NCEO has used a Multi-Attribute Consensus Building process (MACB) (see Vanderwood and Erickson this volume for a detailed description of the process) to create consensus on its national model of outcomes and indicators. Although consensus building appears to be the best practice, outcomes and indicators can be developed by examining the literature and generating new ones or by modifying outcomes and indicators used by others.

STEP 3: ESTABLISH A DATA COLLECTION AND REPORTING SYSTEM

Decide where you will get your data. After the indicators have been selected, the source of data for each indicator must be identified. The best case scenario is to have pre-existing, easily available sources of data for each indicator. Several possible sources and methods for obtaining information are listed in Table 2. Evaluators should ensure that a comprehensive search for data is completed before creating new systems. For those indicators that do not have existing sources, instruments such as an interview or a survey must be developed to collect the information.

Develop/adapt data collection and analysis mechanisms. The collection and analysis of the data for indicators must be completed in a systematic and consistent manner, otherwise the data are useless for making decisions. Efforts must be made to ensure that data are free from significant error and are representative of the student population. NCEO has found that many assessment systems exclude students with disabilities (McGrew, Thurlow, Shriner, & Spiegel, 1992). Decisions based on these systems may be misleading or inappropriate for these students. To prevent this from happening, all students should be included in data collection systems. At the very least, a sampling plan needs to include a representative sample of students with disabilities.

Accommodations or adaptations may be necessary to include students with disabilities in the assessment process. Several differ-

TABLE 2. Possible Sources of Outcomes Data

Data bases/compiled records:

- Attendance, dropout and graduation records
- Budgets
- Club/organization membership lists
- Discipline record
- End of course testing

- Grades
- Portfolio ratings
- School or system-wide test results and national testing
- Student tracking system data

Survey/Interview data from:

- Parent/public
- Policymakers/board members/legislators
- Students

- Staff
- Work-study employers

Individual records:

- Individual student files (e.g., IEP)
- Personnel records
- Therapy notes/records

Other records

- Correspondence files
- Evaluation reports from outside groups
- Minutes of board meetings
- Minutes of PTA meetings

- Observation notes
- Site-based Management Council minutes
- Videotapes: classes, playground, etc.

---

ent types of accommodations can be used without invalidating the results of testing (see Thurlow, Ysseldyke, & Silverstein, 1993 for a complete review of possible accommodations). In some cases an alternative assessment system, such as portfolio analysis, may be necessary to allow all students to participate in the assessment process. Regardless of the assessment method, the key point is to ensure that data are collected from all students on as many of the indicators as possible.

In cases in which new instruments are needed, field testing and examination of the psychometric properties of the instruments are necessary to reduce the amount of error in the data. Educators and special services personnel should connect with evaluation personnel to resolve questions about the adequacy and quality of new measures. The type of analysis conducted with the data depends on the type of comparisons that are desired. Comparisons can be made over time, between groups, or to an absolute standard.

Decide how you will report and use the information. The manner in which the data are reported depends on the original purpose of the assessment and the audiences for which it is intended. Some audiences may want the information in a form that allows them to make decisions about program improvement, others may need the information for accountability purposes. One of the most important decisions to be made deals with the use of the outcomes data. If the data are used in "high stakes" situations, the data invariably will be harder to collect or gain access to the second time around. High stakes exist when individuals or school systems receive rewards or sanctions based on results.

STEP 4: INSTALL THE SYSTEM

Create incentives and support for adoption and use. A system of educational outcomes and indicators cannot be installed without support of the stakeholders affected by it. There are several ways to create support. One, and probably the least desirable, is to use public comparison and sanctions. This creates a high stakes situation. The use of such negative incentives can lead to an overemphasis on appearances, even without substantive change.

Using a combination of positive incentives and technical assistance can be an effective method of installation that does not create a high stakes atmosphere. One way to implement a system is to provide resources, such as test materials, equipment and human resources, to help install the system. A similar incentive is to fund research and demonstration projects to help remove the bugs from the system before turning over to school personnel. Another approach is to help recognize schools that are using an outcomes system and create networks among the schools so that they work together to solve problems. The final, and perhaps most important, method for creating support is to market the system. Through marketing, audiences can become aware of the benefits of an outcomes approach and help stimulate the adoption of the system.

Prepare staff and the public for changes. As part of marketing the system, an effort needs to be made to prepare stakeholders for changes that will occur. Staff and parents will have questions about how they will be affected and may go through a variety of stages from complete lack of concern and awareness to fervent desire to implement the system. Training on the benefits and the mechanics of the process are necessary to reduce resistance and efficiently implement an outcomes model. The advantages of the program should be stressed, while also focusing on the amount of time and effort that will be required to implement the system.

Evaluate the system as it is implemented. The purpose of implementing an outcomes and indicators system is usually to improve some aspect of the educational decision-making process. Evaluation to determine whether the desired change has occurred is essential and should occur through implementation and as long as the system is used. The evaluation questions should be driven by the stated purpose of the outcomes program, and the results should be presented to the staff and public at regular intervals. Special attention should be given to the effect the system has on students with disabilities since many systems exclude these students altogether.

CONCLUSION

An important shift in thinking is occurring in the field of educational reform, moving the focus from the process of education to the results of education. Those involved in making these changes are at the forefront of educational reform and often are attempting to make changes without a model or a set of assumptions on which to rely. The model for change presented here is only one example of a way to move the focus from process to outcomes. We urge others to focus their efforts on moving education to an outcomes focus and to developing methods for establishing this change efficiently and easily.

REFERENCES

Allington, R. L., & McGill-Franzen, A. (1992). Unintended effects of educational reforms in New York. *Educational Policy, 6*(4), 397-414.

McGrew, K. S., Thurlow, M. L., Shriner, J. G., & Spiegel, A.N. (1992). *Inclusion of students with disabilities in national and state data collection programs* (Technical Report 2). Minneapolis: University of Minnesota, National Center on Educational Outcomes.

Thurlow, M. L., Ysseldyke, J. E., & Silverstein, B. (1993). *Testing accommodations for students with disabilities: A review of the literature* (Synthesis Report 4). Minneapolis: University of Minnesota, National Center on Educational Outcomes.

Ysseldyke, J. E., Thurlow, M. L., & Gilman, C. J. (1993a). *Educational outcomes and indicators for early childhood (Age 3).* Minneapolis: University of Minnesota, National Center on Educational Outcomes.

Ysseldyke, J. E., Thurlow, M. L., & Gilman, C. J. (1993b). *Educational outcomes and indicators for early childhood (Age 6).* Minneapolis: University of Minnesota, National Center on Educational Outcomes.

Ysseldyke, J. E., Thurlow, M. L., & Gilman, C. J. (1993c). *Educational outcomes and indicators for individuals at the post-school level.* Minneapolis: University of Minnesota, National Center on Educational Outcomes.

Ysseldyke, J. E., Thurlow, M. L., & Gilman, C. J. (1993d). *Educational outcomes and indicators for students completing school.* Minneapolis: University of Minnesota, National Center on Educational Outcomes.

The Contributions
of Related Services Personnel
to School Reform Efforts

Elizabeth (Bette) Hyde

Puget Sound Educational District
Seattle, Washington

SUMMARY. It is critical in the current climate of rampant educational reform that related services and special education personnel have the skills needed to be a part of all that is happening. This article demonstrates that many of these skills already exist in the rich repertoire of skills of special services and special education personnel. The article also discusses several ways in which some roles can be expanded and skills modified to better meet the needs of schools and students in current educational reforms.

Reform in education is rampant. From Connecticut to Kentucky to California and all points in between, individual states and the federal government are looking at what is not working in public education. Whether speaking of reform or restructuring or paradigm shifting, there seems to be general agreement among public educators and the communities they serve that education needs to be reviewed and redone in some qualitatively different and important ways. While the specifics of reform vary somewhat from state to

Address correspondence to: Elizabeth Hyde, Deputy Superintendent, Puget Sound Educational Service District, 400 SW 152nd Street, Burien, WA 98166-2209.

[Haworth co-indexing entry note]: "The Contributions of Related Services Personnel to School Reform Efforts." Hyde, Elizabeth (Bette). Co-published simultaneously in *Special Services in the Schools* (The Haworth Press, Inc.) Vol. 9, No. 2, 1994, pp. 127-138; and: *Educational Outcomes for Students with Disabilities* (ed: James E. Ysseldyke, and Martha L. Thurlow) The Haworth Press, Inc., 1994, pp. 127-138. Multiple copies of this article/chapter may be purchased from The Haworth Document Delivery Center [1-800-3-HAWORTH; 9:00 a.m. - 5:00 p.m. (EST)].

state and site to site, there are several recurrent themes. There is typically an increased emphasis on accountability for students' learning, for teachers' instructional strategies, indeed, entire school sites (State of Washington, 1993). There is a greater involvement of others in education, including private corporations, social service agencies, student and parents involved in site-based teams, and the entire Cities and Communities in School movement (Cities in Schools, 1993). Relatedly, there is a heightened demand for schools to effectively and clearly communicate with their publics. These communications include schools' mission, short and long term goals, specific student achievements, and long range plans–all in jargon free terms.

In this climate of educational reform, the skills and the roles of related service in special education personnel are critical. These skills are obviously important in the provision and oversight of services to students with disabilities. The skills take the form of diagnostic/prescriptive expertise in student programming. In the area of educational reform, however, related services personnel may be required to advance a new type of advocacy for students with disabilities. For example, in the context of expanded site-based teams, issues of confidentiality and need-to-know communications become paramount. Similarly, with increased emphasis on accountability and a shift from the unit of measure being individual students to individual school sites, there could be subtle and not so subtle pressures to not include the performances of students with disabilities. The important roles of related services personnel in producing and advocating for students with disabilities is well documented throughout this volume.

The emphasis here, however, will be on the role of related service personnel in system reform. The basic tenet of this article is that the skills of related services staff will serve them well in the educational reform movement. The same diagnostic-prescriptive, accountability-based, communicative skills that have been the "bread and butter" of the school psychologist and other related services personnel will be critical in producing needed change. These staff need to shift their focus from the individual child to the system as a whole and apply the same skills to this larger entity. Since these skills are second nature, this article makes them explicit so that they might be applied to the diagnosis and remediation of the total system. What follows is a list of selected components of educational reform and suggestions and examples of new roles that related service personnel can contribute.

ASSESSMENT

Assessment is tantamount in educational reform. Reform calls for more and/or different assessments, by different teams of individuals, using different measures. There is a call for "authentic assessment" in terms of national, state, and locally developed goals in a variety of academic and interpersonal/citizenship arenas. The demands of the individualized education program and the legal requirements for assessment/reassessment have made assessment an ongoing industry. What remains is for related services personnel to apply these assessment skills to the system. That is, the same task analysis skills that have served them well in student diagnosis can be used to dissect the component skills needed for system reform and system health. Task analysis works well, whether one is applying it to diagnosing steps toward mastery of a classroom task or the communication needs of a site-based team. Similarly, one can task analyze the steps needed in a school building's strategic plan and steps required to involve and engage the public in the implementation of this plan. Support staff can model this type of task analytic thinking and teach it to other building members as they go about the task of examining and rebuilding their educational system. The direct instruction literature is replete with examples of dissecting and sequencing the component parts of the task so that you can see the composite results.

Simple observational skills are an extremely important weapon in the assessment arsenal. In the hustle of reform, it is important to step back and observe objectively and openly what is occurring. Instead of applying these observational skills to a child in the classroom, related services personnel can apply these same skills to the function of a site-based team, to student responses to a proposed curriculum adjustment, and to the reaction of communities to school communications. Again, it is important not just that the related services personnel perform these observational skills, but that they also teach others to do so. Simply listening and objectively recording the reactions of staff and students can assist in assessing the status of the educational reform and altering its course accordingly. Related services staff can provide a variety of simple, easy-to-use recording formats, so that progress can be observed and documented and decisions can be based, at least in part, on data.

The training of related services staff in assessment typically includes a strong background in measurement theory. This needs to be applied to educational reform efforts. Simple measurement concepts such as validity, reliability, and sampling can greatly assist and strengthen educational reform efforts. Despite the urgency to develop system-wide performance measures, these measures must have some validity across more than one classroom setting and some reliability across more than one instructor. Here a simple introductory level discussion of measurements theory could save embarrassment and strengthen reform. An important measurement concept that seems frequently overlooked is that of sampling. If a school or school system wants to assess educational reform progress to date, there is no need to measure all students/families. A more economical approach would be to sample a random or stratified part of the group to determine progress in a more efficient and cost effective fashion. Related services personnel can assist with sampling design. They can train building staff in how to create this design.

Educational reform typically calls not only for academic goals but also for other interpersonal or life skills goals as well. Such interpersonal and life skill changes have been historically the realm of related services personnel, including school psychologists, school counselors, occupational/physical therapists, etc. These interpersonal measures are typically not pathology oriented and might include such favorites as maturity measures, sociograms, and "climate" assessments. There is a related movement throughout many states in social services reform utilizing real life authentic outcomes. Rather than document numbers of trainings and meetings, social service reformers are demanding to know what real life changes occur in people's day to day lives. Here, related services personnel can assist in designing reliable ways of documenting and gathering these outcomes.

ACCOUNTABILITY

Assessment as a element of educational reform is closely tied to the second critical element of reform accountability. Assessment is often undertaken to collect accountability data. Related services staff have some very specialized and pertinent skills to offer to accountability programs. First, they seem to be more comfortable than most school personnel with educational laws. Related services personnel have experience in reading, dissecting, and interpreting laws pertaining to children with a variety of special needs, including eligibility for Special Education, Chapter I, and/or Gifted and Talented services. This experience with laws results in most related service personnel realizing that the intent behind such laws is to benefit students. Consequently, laws are interpreted from a "reasonable person's" perspective and not from a fear of legal language or minutia. The same appreciation and non-aversion for the law can be applied to state and federal educational reform efforts to assist staffs in interpreting and implementing these laws. Second, as discussed above, related services personnel come to the reform effort with a diagnostic-prescriptive mindset. This mindset can be applied not just to children and families but to staff relationships, school climate, and the law. The task is always simple–discerning component parts, and building back a better whole.

A similar type of mindset of equal importance is the all-children-can-learn mindset. While many school staff verbalize and support this mindset, related services personnel live it. Part of the diagnostic process is looking for not just needs but also relative strengths on which to build. Increasingly social service research is replete with individuals talking about the "half full model" and assessment tools to document strengths (McKnight, 1987). School nurses and other health related service providers are well aware of the Healthy Communities effort that is part of the World Health Organization (DeLeeuw & Goumans, 1993). Throughout the world, cities and communities are collaborating to define the indicators of community strengths that are valued and sought. Related services personnel can assist school sites in making explicit healthy indicators that classroom, school sites, and communities seek for children and their families. Accounting for school strengths as well as school needs would seem a critical component for an effective and visionary educational reform.

A critical component of accountability is communicating the findings. In some states (State of Washington, 1993) state law dictates what results will be communicated to whom and how. There is increased emphasis on communicating in a clear, meaningful fashion, not only individual student results but also the profiles of buildings and entire district's relative performance compared to other school buildings and other school districts. Everyone likes telling others good news; however, in a climate of reform, not every effort is bound to be successful. Related services personnel have experience communicating low ability test scores, limited adaptive potentials, and guarded prognosis. They know the importance of clearly, directly, and supportively communicating negative data.

Educational reform demands honesty and directness in communicating the results of reform efforts. Here again, related services personnel can assist in designing and delivering classroom, building, or district-wide data. Often such relatively negative results mobilize the community and result in far more positive findings in the long run. Finally in terms of communication skills, related services personnel bring one additional talent. Particularly among partners new at teaming, there is a tendency to "go on and on." Related services personnel typically communicate results in a task-oriented fashion. That is, their job is to communicate their findings and recommendations with the parents, with the team, and with the student him/herself. Consequently, communications are typically well-timed, well-orchestrated, and well-delivered. This type of orientation to tasks can do wonders to facilitate struggling site-based teams, help parent conferences move along, or intervene in some hostile moments of a community meeting.

EXTENDED TEAM

A third common element of educational reform is that of an extended team. Not only are there different assessments to assure greater accountability, but there are also more to whom the schools are accountable and with whom they are teaming to achieve reform. Increasingly, "outsiders" are being welcomed into the school team.

More and more social service agencies are "co-locating" in school buildings. Related services personnel can assist with this interface by helping to interpret the professional jargon on both sides. Typically related services personnel are more familiar than most other educators with social service jargon. Related services personnel, consequently, can serve as a bridge to translate and ultimately reduce the use of jargon by both social service providers and educators. In this era of educational reform, the agencies that are included are not only the typical social service agencies but also juvenile justice, local police units, and sometimes private service providers. In this increased "mixture" of personnel, issues of confidentiality are accentuated. Related services personnel are, again, the school employees most familiar with the Family Rights and Privacy Act and nuances of confidential communication. In these new collaborations, all sides are typically a little nervous at the onset. Related services personnel can model and help to set a tone of cooperation and effective ground rules for schools and agencies interactions.

This extended team also includes greater parent involvement. The involvement is "greater" in the sense that more parents are involved and each of them may have more in-depth involvement. While increased parent involvement is almost as sacred as apple pie, many very good educators are not quite ready. There is something deceptively simple about the term "parent involvement." Parent involvement ranges from signing a typed IEP, or discussing what a child might need, to being an equal partner at the table when the design of the assessment is being brainstormed. A major tenet of current thinking in educational reform is to have parents as "real," equal partners. In this context, related services personnel can play a large role. This role includes communicating and modeling how to effectively partner with parents, being there when the process breaks down, and providing assistance with a few staff who feel this equality is not for them. Assistance could come in the form of one-on-one support, classes for faculty, discussion groups, and or direct instruction and coaching in communication techniques.

Educational reform also calls for greater student involvement. Student involvement varies with different sites, but typically students from primary grades through high school can be involved in site-based teams and/or in determining their own individual goals for learning. Generally, related services personnel have more training and experience in one-on-one communications with students. These staff can provide valuable insights, consultation, and training to teachers and administrators in how to solicit meaningful student communication and genuine involvement. Proponents of service learning and/or democratic schools would argue that such meaningful student involvement is a prerequisite for truly effective educational reform (Howard & Kenny, 1992).

A major illustration of this element of extended team is site-based decision making. While state laws may not call for site-based teams per se, the participatory and inclusive nature of educational reform certainly points to the need for more accountability and "empowerment" (Glickman, 1992) at the building site. As Glickman points out, site-based decision making is deceptively simple. The tendency to throw together selected teams of individuals and expect them to make important decisions almost inevitably leads to problems. By contrast, clearly defined site-based decisions over time yield powerful effects for staff and students (Glickman, 1990). In this site-based context, related services staff bring much needed skills. First, related services staff–particularly school psychologists, counselors, and social workers–have expertise and training in group facilitation. Getting a group to get started takes skill and time. Establishing clear ground rules for group membership, operating principles, and a clear listing of the expectations and requirements for the group all help to prevent misunderstandings and inefficient use of time. Related services can help with getting the group started and keeping it on task. Training in group dynamics and team building can be useful when the site team falters, when new members join, and/or assignments and expectations change. It is critical that related services personnel model these skills and teach others to model them. Particularly in the context of site-based decision making, the principal is an important "student" of related services personnel.

The ability to listen is critical for all players in site-based decision making (Hoyle, 1992). While most of us advocate and profess to have fine listening skills, it is important that these skills be applied in an ongoing manner to site-based teaming. Related services staff can provide a workshop in listening skills and methods to improve listening to others. Many instances of site-based decision making difficulties are attributable ultimately to the team not taking the time to find out exactly what was the problem, but rather presuming they knew. To listen openly, to reserve judgment or answer, and to attend to others' points of view can do a great deal to shift paradigms and perspectives and alter the system. An effective way to instruct others about listening skills is to model do's and don'ts. The comedy inherent in these contrasts helps make the lessons "stick."

There will be conflicts in the area of site-based decision making skills. As Glickman (1990) points out, one of the paradoxes of site-based decision making is that the more genuine the process, the harder it gets. Related services personnel have expertise in conflict resolution and can assist with the conflicts that will (and probably should) occur. In most school districts related services personnel are *not* site-based but rather serve more than one building. Consequently, these individuals are in an excellent position to provide expertise without getting caught up in a process. Indeed probably the best investment of the time of related services personnel for educational reform is at the site level. The same diagnostic/prescriptive, observational, and inclusion skills that related services staff typically apply to students can be well adapted to support and enhance the efforts of the site building team per se.

PROGRAM EVALUATION

Educational reform demands increased accountability by program, by school, and by district. Related services personnel bring specific skills in the arena of program evaluation. First, related services personnel can provide invaluable data for describing the school site. Health personnel typically have access to county and/or health demographics that can describe the current school as well as provide past and future trend data about the site and its neighborhoods. School social workers and school psychologists can provide data about school building and school classroom climate as well as student and community perception of school needs and strengths. School language specialists can assist with school climate assessments by looking at connotative descriptors and meaning that people apply to their school buildings. All these data serve as a good base line measure by which to examine the effectiveness of school reform interventions.

Second, related services personnel typically come with knowledge of psychoeducational school literature. These staff can bring to the building site research and best practices in educational reform. For example, simply knowing that the literature speaks of paradoxes and talks of problems that will occur in site-based decision making may help a site through some difficult times. Pooling the psychoeducational literature routinely read by the team of related services personnel can greatly assist the school site in using data to design programs.

Third, related services personnel can assist with the design of a program evaluation. Simple as it sounds, many sites do not define what they are going to evaluate ahead of time. Rather, contrary to the cardinal rule, reform is implemented without any kind of base line measures of what one hopes to change. Related services personnel can assist by being a voice stressing the importance of premeasures and helping to design a system by which premeasures will be sampled over a period of time. Educational reform calls for improvement not only in academics but also citizenship. Many seemingly easy measures of school citizenship and involvement become problematic when examined. For example, does number of absences or number of tardies mean the same thing across classrooms and across schools? Similarly, "disciplinary referrals" can be applied to quite different behaviors in different classrooms and different schools. To really measure the effectiveness of change, it is important to have common definitions for these seemingly simple terms ahead of time and throughout. Related services staff can prove valuable assistance in helping a teacher and/or an entire site define and measure these terms.

In the context of program evaluation, related services personnel can offer their skills in grantsmanship. Throughout the country, it is highly unusual to have all the financial resources seemingly simple terms ahead of time and throughout. Related services staff can provide valuable assistance in helping a teacher and/or an entire site define and measure these terms.

In the context of program evaluation, related services personnel can offer their skills in grantsmanship. Throughout the country, it is highly unusual to have all the financial resources available to each school site to do the kind of job they want to as part of educational reform. Typically, school teachers, school and school sites find themselves in the unenviable position of seeking "external funding opportunities." External funding opportunities come in a variety of packages, ranging from the federal government to district level mini-grants to neighborhood contributions. To secure external funding, there is typically some type of grant proposal required. The grantsmanship work that related services personnel staff typically do in terms of assisting with Chapter I applications, special education/special needs grants, or their own work in securing a MA or PhD all set the standard for what most grants require. A simple one page descriptor of the need, goal/objectives, and measures used typically suffices. Related services staff can either write such grant proposals or, better still, engage both students and staff in proposal creation.

CONCLUSION

Related services staff bring a rich repertoire of skills to facilitate and enhance educational reform. The skills of assessment and accountability so critical in the individual IEP process can be applied to developing individualized educational plans for classrooms or for schools. The listening, observational, diagnostic/prescriptive, and remedial programming skills of related services personnel can be applied to both the student and the system. These staff's skills in team building, group facilitation, and meaningful involvement of students, parents, and communities will serve them well whether programming for students or reforming the system. Indeed, the whole definition of "related services" in federal legislation is that of providing services necessary for students to receive and benefit from the free appropriate publication education. It could be argued that the same skills, transferred from the student focus to a system focus, similarly enable all students to acquire not only an appropriate but improved public education.

REFERENCES

Cities in Schools: Students celebrate new partnership. (1993, December 8). *The Seattle Times.*

DeLeeuw, E. & Goumas, M. (1993, December 10). *Current research and evaluation of Healthy Cities Programs.* Paper presented at the International Healthy Cities and Communities Conference, San Francisco, CA.

Glickman, C. D. (1990). Pushing school reform to a new edge: The seven ironies of school empowerment. *Phi Delta Kappan, 72*(1), pp. 68-75.

Glickman, C. D. (1992). The essence of school reform: the prose has begun. *Educational Leadership, 50*(1), pp. 24-27.

Howard, R. & Kenny, R. (1992). Education for democracy: promoting citizenship and critical reasoning through school governance. In A. Garrod (Ed.), *Learning for a lifetime: Moral education in perspective and practice.* New York: Praeger Press.

Hoyle, J. R. (1992, November). Ten commandments for successful sited-based management. *NASSP Bulletin, 76*(547), pp. 81-87.

McKnight, J. L. (1987, June). *The future of low-income neighborhoods and the people who reside there: A capacity-oriented strategy for neighborhood development.* Evenston, IL: Northwestern University, Matt Foundation, Center for Urban Affairs and Policy Research.

State of Washington, House of Representatives, 53rd Legislature, Regular Session. Education Reform, ESHB §1209, pp. 1-35, (1993).

Broadening Educational Outcomes Beyond Academics

James G. Shriner

Clemson University

SUMMARY. Current educational reform activities are stressing academic achievement, generally at the expense of excluding other, nonacademic outcomes. For students with disabilities, as well as other special needs students, nonacademic outcomes are considered essential. In this article, the ways in which nonacademic outcomes have been identified as important are described (through model development, in national data collection programs, and in states). The author discusses issues related to the measurement of nonacademic outcomes, then concludes with issues and recommendations relevant for special services personnel.

Voluntary national . . . standards should not address nonacademic areas such as student values, beliefs, attitudes and behaviors. (National Education Goals Panel, 1993, p. 6)

"Higher standards" and "better educational results" are common rallying cries heard in schools, district offices, state education agencies and national policy-planning meetings. Goals 2000: Educate America Act (P.L. 103-227) has been signed into law, begin-

Address correspondence to: James G. Shriner, 400 Tillman Hall, Department of Elementary and Secondary Education, Clemson University, Clemson, SC 29634-0709.

[Haworth co-indexing entry note]: "Broadening Educational Outcomes Beyond Academics." Shriner, James G. Co-published simultaneously in *Special Services in the Schools* (The Haworth Press, Inc.) Vol. 9, No. 2, 1994, pp. 139-154; and: *Educational Outcomes for Students with Disabilities* (ed: James E. Ysseldyke, and Martha L. Thurlow) The Haworth Press, Inc., 1994, pp. 139-154. Multiple copies of this article/chapter may be purchased from The Haworth Document Delivery Center [1-800-3-HAWORTH; 9:00 a.m. - 5:00 p.m. (EST)].

139

ning a chain reaction of standards-setting, preparation of curricular frameworks, and development of newer, performance-based assessments. The eight National Education Goals are the focal point of Goals 2000. These goals set the course for long-term reform efforts that are to improve the educational system (see Ysseldyke and Thurlow, Table 1 this volume, for a list of the National Education Goals). They span the educational lifetime of children, youth and adults–from preschool readiness to adult literacy. They also cover the academic, employability and citizenship, health and discipline, and socio/emotional development and deportment of the children, teachers, and parents who make up the educational community.

Tremendous efforts have been focused on academic goals largely

TABLE 1. Nonacademic Domains and Outcomes of the NCEO Model

Physical Health

- Makes healthy lifestyle choices
- Is aware of basic safety, fitness, and health care needs

Responsibility and Independence

- Gets about in the environment
- Is responsible for self

Contribution and Citizenship

- Demonstrates compliance with school-community rules
- Knowledge of significance of voting and procedures necessary to register and vote
- Volunteerism

Personal and Social Adjustment

- Copes effectively with personal challenges, frustrations, and stressors
- Has a good self image
- Respects cultural/individual differences
- Gets along with other people

Satisfaction

- Student satisfaction with school experience
- Parent/guardian satisfaction with the education that students receive
- Community satisfaction with the education that students receive

because of the perceptions that America's position in the global marketplace is weakening and that without a dramatically improved workforce the slippage is likely to continue (Porter, 1993). There are federally funded standards-setting activities in all of the academic areas. Most of these projects are preparing *content standards,* which define what students should know and be able to do in the subject area, and *performance standards,* which help define how good is good enough on assessments of progress toward the content standards (Selden, 1992). Additionally, some of these groups are addressing the issue of opportunity-to-learn (OTL) standards that are part of Goals 2000.

Assessment becomes an integral part of operationalizing the standards rhetoric. It is sometimes argued that assessments drive the curriculum–what gets measured, gets taught (Leone, McLaughlin, & Meisel, 1992). If this premise is true, is it possible that some very important educational outcomes are being ignored? The answer is–yes *and* no. As exemplified by the opening quotation of this article, Washington officials do not want to stray from an intense focus on academics. Even when assessments of non-academic outcomes (e.g., health, workskills) are endorsed by the National Education Goals Panel, they will not be defined as essential elements of any accountability or evaluation system (M. Orland, personal communication, December 2, 1993). This is because the Goals Panel leadership believes that national content and performance standards should address only those areas listed in Goal 3, academic goals.

However, there are national and state efforts that seek to strengthen the broader educational experience for students. For example, the Department of Labor has published a report calling for instruction and assessment efforts to include students' basic skills, thinking skills and personal qualities (Secretary's Commission on Achieving Necessary Skills, 1992). The American Public Welfare Association identified the outcome areas of physical health and safety, social/emotional, cognitive/academic and productivity/employment (American Public Welfare Association, 1991). As an example of states' activities, Michigan has initiated a student Employability Skills Portfolio to document each pupil's academic, personal management, and teamwork skills (Stemmer, Brown, & Smith, 1992). The Employability Portfolios were introduced because leaders from business and industry needed documentation that exiting students were competent academically and personally. Students who know a great deal but fail to take care of themselves or show up for work are not wise investment risks. "Helping all students learn the skills they'll need for the workplace is . . . an economic necessity" (O'Neil, 1992).

So, we are left with some uncertainty about the important results of schooling. Yet, for many special services providers, it is not so confusing an issue. Students who receive special services are included in the group referred to as the "forgotten half" of the school population, those who possibly will not enter postsecondary education (O'Neil, 1992). One national effort that focuses on education outcomes for all students, including students with special needs, is the National Center on Education Outcomes (NCEO). Using a cross-section of stakeholders, a model was developed that included domains beyond academics, such as physical health, responsibility and independence, contribution and citizenship, academic and functional literacy, personal and social adjustment and satisfaction (see Ysseldyke & Thurlow, in this volume).

The non-academic domains of the NCEO model serve as focal points for the remainder of this article. The outcomes within each of these domains are shown in Table 1. Particular attention is paid to these because students who receive special services in the schools are usually in most need of instruction in these areas (Winget, 1994). Consider, for example, students with behavioral disorders who receive special education services. The NCEO domains of Responsibility and Independence and Personal and Social Adjustment constitute the critical core of educational programs for these students (Peacock Hill Working Group, 1991). Indeed, academic standards and outcomes only provide a partial picture of the purposes of schooling, and at least one major report places personal/social behavioral characteristics as a higher priority for the success of educational reform than academic gains (Carson, Huelskamp, & Woodall, 1992).

DATA FROM NATIONAL PROGRAMS

One of the activities of the NCEO is the secondary analysis of national and state data bases to describe the functional characteristics of students with disabilities in the current reform-oriented environment. McGrew, Spiegel, Thurlow, and Kim (1994) subsequently evaluated 13 data bases by mapping the variables contained in each to the conceptual model developed by NCEO. Table 2 is a matrix of these data bases and the nonacademic domains of the NCEO model relevant to this article. Ten of the data bases were identified as having potentially useful information for the nonacademic domains of the model. The domain of Responsibility and Independence was most often represented (eight data bases), whereas Satisfaction information occurred in only two data sets.

Despite the number of data bases collecting information on nonacademic domains, we still lack data on these outcomes for students with disabilities. There is considerable exclusion of students with disabilities from national assessment and data collection programs (McGrew, Thurlow, Shriner, & Spiegel, 1992). The excluded percentage is estimated to be as high as 40% to 50% for educational data sets (e.g., National Assessment of Educational Progress), but is somewhat lower in noneducational efforts (e.g., National Health Interview Survey). Also, there is significant variability in both the terminology used to identify students in these data bases, and in the grouping of categories of students who receive special services in the schools (McGrew, Algozzine, Spiegel, Thurlow, & Ysseldyke, 1993). It is very difficult to be certain about the specific characteristics of students included in these data bases. Strategies for addressing these issues for *all* students are needed.

STATES' NONACADEMIC OUTCOMES

NCEO has routinely sought information from states about the outcomes they specified for students with and without disabilities, and about their assessment efforts in both academic and nonacademic domains. As part of a survey (Shriner & Thurlow, 1992), states were asked to provide their formal, written statements of outcomes. Documents were received from 17 states, and these were mapped to the domains in the NCEO model (see Table 1 for list of domains and outcomes). Table 3 is the matrix of all nonacademic domains in the NCEO model and the number of state outcomes for each.

TABLE 2. NCEO Nonacademic Domains Included in National Data Bases

DOMAIN	DATA SET												
	CPS	HSTS	MF	NAEP	NALS	NCS	NELS	NHES	NHIS	NHSDA	NLTS	NSFG	YRBS
Physical Health			X				X		X	X	X		X
Responsibility and Independence			X		X		X	X	X		X	X	X
Contribution and Citizenship			X		X		X			X	X		
Personal and Social Adjustment			X	X			X				X		X
Satisfaction			X				X						

CPS = Current Population Survey (1993)
HSTS = High School Transcript Study (1990)
MF = Monitoring the Future (1993)
NAEP = National Assessment of Educational Progress (1992)
NALS = National Adult Literacy Survey (1992)
NCS = National Crime Survey (1989)
NLTS = National Longitudinal Transition Study (1987)

NELS = National Education Longitudinal Survey (1992)
NHES = National Household Education Survey (1991)
NHIS = National Health Interview Survey (1988)
NHSDA = National Household Survey of Drug Abuse (1993)
NSFG = National Survey of Family Growth (1988)
YRBS = Youth Risk Behavior Survey (1993)

TABLE 3. Number of States' Goals by NCEO Nonacademic Domains

States

NCEO DOMAINS	AR	CO	FL	GA	HI	IN	KS	KY	LA	MI	MN	NH	NM	NY	TX	VT	VA
Physical Health	1		1	1	2	2	3	6		14			3	3		1	1
Responsibility and Independence	8		7	4	5	8		6		31	8	2	4	8		3	
Contribution and Citizenship	2		2	1	3	1	1	2		3	3		1	3		3	
Personal and Social Adjustment	14		12	6	2	3	6	14		13	8	3	2	15		17	1
Satisfaction						14									4		

145

It is clear that states do place some importance on outcomes of schooling other than academics. All but two states had outcomes that matched the nonacademic domains of the NCEO model. Also, there appears to be some degree of representation across all domains *except* Satisfaction. Only Indiana and Texas clearly listed Satisfaction outcomes for their students. Responsibility and Independence and Personal and Social Adjustment are generally the most frequently observed domain areas across all states. The high number of objectives in these domains for the state of Michigan reflects its approach of defining separate outcomes for each category of exceptionality served in the state. Still, these data suggest that students' social development and behavior may be more than a minor focus of their instructional experiences regardless of where they reside.

MEASUREMENT OF NONACADEMIC OUTCOMES

Even if states list nonacademic goals and outcomes for students, what is known about student progress toward them? Two sources of information collected by NCEO indicate what the states actually do to measure these outcomes. The first evidence comes from the annual surveys of states. States were asked about the nonacademic domains for which they conducted a statewide assessment effort. Figure 1 shows the number of states that collected data across a three-year period for the areas of post-school status, vocational skills, functional life skills, and attitudes.

Almost half the states conduct some kind of post-school follow-up measure. Often, these efforts were part of federally-funded research or evaluation projects (Shriner, Bruininks, Deno, McGrew, Thurlow, & Ysseldyke, 1991). Fewer states, however, reported that they conduct assessments of vocational and functional skills, or student attitudes about schooling. There is a *minor* upward trend in these efforts, some of which may be due to a greater interest in nonacademic outcomes.

The second source of evidence about states' measurement activities in these areas comes from an additional survey conducted by Ysseldyke, Vanderwood, and Reschly (1993). These researchers asked state data managers about the availability and accessibility of data in their states' data bases for the NCEO conceptual model of

FIGURE 1. Number of States Collecting Nonacademic Data over Three
Years

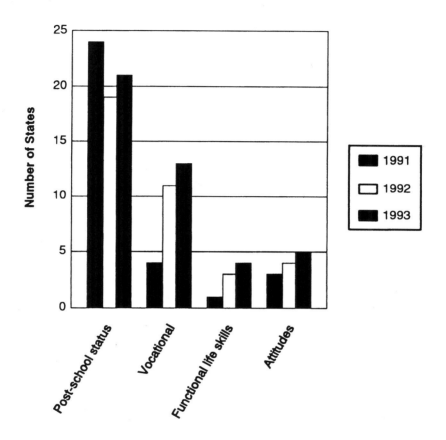

outcomes and indicators. The data managers were asked to rate the
data on a scale ranging from "the data could never be made available" to "the data are currently collected and reported at the state
level." Selected results from this survey for nonacademic areas are
shown in Table 4.

Thirteen states indicated that data on the degree to which students complied with school and community rules were readily
available and accessible in their data bases. These data are most
often suspension and expulsion information that are reported to the

TABLE 4. States with Available Data on NCEO Outcomes

Domain	Outcome	States
Physical Health	Makes healthy lifestyle choices	AR, DC, IA, MN, WV
	Is aware of basic safety, fitness, and health care needs	DC, IL
	Is physically fit	RI
Responsibility & Independence	Gets about in the environment	DC, MI, TX
	Is responsible for self	---
Contribution & Citizenship	Complies with school and community rules	AR, CA, DC, FL, IL, KY, MA, MN, NC, NM, OH, SC, TN
	Knows significance of voting and procedures to register to vote	AR, MI
	Volunteers	DC, MI
Personal/Social Adjustment	Copes with frustration and stress	IL, KY
	Has good self image	KY, MN
	Gets along with other people	DC, KY, MI
	Respects cultural & individual differences	DC, KY
Satisfaction	Student satisfaction with school	DE, MI, MD
	Parent/guardian satisfaction with education students received	DE, MI
	Community satisfaction with education students received	DC, DE, MI

state (M. Vanderwood, personal communication, July 7, 1994). No more than five states could report on any of the other nonacademic outcomes. What is most interesting, is that although the nonacademic domains of "responsibility and independence" and "personal and social adjustment" had been the most likely for states to include in their written outcomes, only six states have data available related to any outcome within those domains. No state collects and reports data on the outcome of "Is responsible for self," and only

Kentucky can report on all four outcomes within the domain of Personal and Social Adjustment. Satisfaction data are part of the current efforts in only four states. Ysseldyke, Vanderwood, and Reschly (1993) indicated that most nonacademic data are not, and most likely would not be, part of statewide measurement efforts.

ISSUES AND RECOMMENDATIONS FOR SPECIAL SERVICES PERSONNEL

It appears that instruction and assessment related to the nonacademic outcomes of schooling are enigmatic issues for professionals at most levels of the educational system. Some national and state efforts stress the importance of addressing both physical and social emotional development, whereas others strongly recommend avoiding the issue altogether (cf. National Education Goals Panel, 1993). Even among those states that list nonacademic results among their formal goals of schooling, there is far less emphasis given to measuring the extent to which these results have been obtained. Several concerns and issues can be raised about these findings.

Addressing the current situation. Special services personnel deal with the nonacademic aspects of childrens' school experiences more often than most other professionals. Thus, it is important for those providing special services to be informed participants in local and state activities related to the definition, instruction, and assessment of those nonacademic results believed to be important for the long-term life success of *all* students. Getting multiple perspectives from special services personnel in local discussions of outcomes helps ensure that a broader community understands and supports those school outcomes for which resources are to be allocated. Interagency cooperation in these efforts should be encouraged. Guetzloe (1993) noted that an "expanded program of interagency communication and collaboration [is needed] to advocate for children and youth" (p. 306). The viewpoints of persons familiar with students who have a variety of special services needs will help avoid the situation about which Leone et al. (1992) issued this warning:

Agendas that address only academic outcomes are incomplete. If . . . other aspects of learning are dismissed as inappropriate and inconsequential, many youngsters in special education will be shortchanged and all students will miss a vital part of schooling. (p. 12)

These authors were warning about assessment-driven instruction, but a complete overhaul of the data collection and assessment system is *not* warranted. Data do exist on the nonacademic skills and functioning of students in many states, but they are "buried" in the larger set of general education assessment information (Shriner, Ysseldyke, Thurlow, & Honetschlager, 1994). Special services personnel should encourage local and state data managers and administrators to take a closer look at what *is* known about how students are faring in areas like physical health, responsibility and independence and social and personal adjustment. Examination of existing data may bolster additional activities in these areas.

Teaching/assessing basic processes. Of the nonacademic domains, those related to social/behavioral outcomes have received some not-so-pleasant attention in recent years. Several national studies on student behavior and violence in schools presented an alarming picture of what students who receive special services experience and perceive as their daily environment in the education system. The American Psychological Association's Commission on Violence and Youth reported that children with disabilities are placed at risk for violent victimization more often than the general population. Often, this was because they had not been taught social or self-advocacy skills (American Psychological Association, 1993). The percent of students, by social group, perceived as likely victims of abuse or violence in schools was 65% for "social outcasts" or "weaklings"; 48% for "trouble-makers"; and 31% for students with disabilities (Leitman & Binns, 1993). The superintendent of a major urban school district recently commented on these types of findings by stating: "students who are afraid . . . can't learn [because of] the fear they experience in school" (Hotakainen, 1994, p. 2B).

It is no surprise that students' behavior is often a barrier to learning and achievement, and undermines many innovative, promising efforts and practices. There are consistent calls from within education and from business to directly confront and alleviate disruptive, antisocial behavior and to teach students those skills they need to negotiate the real world (Huml, 1994). The missing portions of students' education, according to many in the field, are social/behavioral skills and competencies that make academic learning more likely—especially for students experiencing behavioral or learning difficulties (Peacock Hill Working Group, 1991). Huml (1994) listed many basic processes that may be necessary components of students' school experience, including: listening, following directions, dealing with pressures, problem solving, dealing with anger, and accepting consequences. This list might have included negotiation skills, and are arguably the very cornerstones of success in early life. Special services providers already do some teaching of these skills, but it is clear that many students are in need of such instruction if schools are to be places that are conducive to learning (National Goal 7). As Huml (1994) questioned, "Isn't it assumed by a previous national effort to teach children to 'just say no!' that basic training in social interaction and personal responsibility have occurred?" Just as some students need direct instruction in basic reading skills, others will require similar experiences if they are to learn decision making and self-control. This is not to say that school is the only place where these skills could or should be taught. In on-the-job experience or vocational programs and community settings, all of these competencies can be applied in real-world, authentic situations, and assessed through genuine performance-based measures. This is the best intervention-assessment link available—where accomplishment may mean the difference between more time in the judicial system or the educational system. These systems are not always equally accessible to students who lack social-behavioral skills.

Expect resistance and plan for controversy. Rosenberg, Wilson, Maheady, and Sindelar (1992) argued that:

> The importance of direct-social-skills training for students who do not readily learn indirectly or who have inadvertently learned inappropriate social responses cannot be overstated. A much greater emphasis must be placed on the development of programs that foster and maintain prosocial behavior. (p. 416)

These same arguments can be made for personal care and responsibility skills (American Public Welfare Association, 1992). But, there is a strong reluctance to include nonacademic skills in reform-oriented instruction and assessment systems. As the National Education Goals Panel position statement makes clear, even if measures of nonacademic skills are endorsed by the Panel, they will not be included in any accountability efforts. States, too, are avoiding or deferring all decisions to measure nonacademic outcomes at this time. This is especially true in states that have already begun to seek outcomes-based-accountability data (J. Haigh, personal communication, December 2, 1993). Why is this so? Mostly because of the vociferous outcry over states' outcomes statements that deal with personal care/social and behavioral skills as well as academics (Consortium for Policy Research in Education, 1993). It is really *not* the measurement of nonacademic results that causes concern, it is the perceived overstepping of the role of schools in society. Harold and Maples (1992) pointed out that in Pennsylvania the views of conservative social groups were expressed with such intensity that the State Department of Education rejected its initial decision to include personal care, attitudes toward self and others, and social/interpersonal skills as the important outcomes of education for the states' students. Writing about the conservative position, Hoge (1993) explained that measurement of appropriate personal and behavioral competencies was *not* an appropriate activity for schools.

CONCLUSION

Special services providers at all levels can expect to face the issues surrounding nonacademic outcomes. The concern is that avoidance of assessment may mean a significant diversion of resources away from programs that deal with these skills (Shriner, in press). As one state's former Commissioner of Education said, "For those who want to advance a results oriented, data-based decision making and policy system, it is best to avoid the inclusion or reporting of such information in state plans" (G. Mammenga, personal communication, April 10, 1993). It is likely to be extremely difficult to win legislative and financial support for any set of state goals that address desired student attitudes and behaviors. The belief is that schools should stick to academics because a well-educated student body will take care of personal, social, community, and environmental interactions just as their parents did (OBE, 1994). There are two questions that special services personnel must ask themselves. First, do they believe this is a likely scenario for today's students? Second, is relying on such an approach the best way to address the needs of the students they see every day?

REFERENCES

American Psychological Association. (1993). *Violence & Youth: Psychology's response.* New York: Commission on Violence and Youth.

American Public Welfare Association. (1991). *Joining forces.* Washington, DC: Council of Chief State School Officers.

Carson, C. C., Huelskamp, R. M., & Woodall, T. D. (1992). *Perspectives on education in America.* Albuquerque, NM: Sandia National Laboratories.

Consortium for Policy Research in Education. (1993). *Developing content standards: Creating a process for change.* New Brunswick, NJ: CPRE Policy Briefs.

Guetzloe, E. C. (1993). The special education initiative: Responding to changing problems, populations, and paradigms. *Behavioral Disorders, 18,* 303-307.

Harold, G., & Maples, K. (1992). Perspectives on the future. *Teaching Exceptional Children, 25*(1), 43.

Hoge, A. (1993, November 10). How do you measure that outcome? *Education Week,* p. 25.

Hotakainen, R. (1994, July 9). Report: Student behavior a barrier. *Minneapolis Star-Tribune,* p. 2B.

Huml, F. J. (1994, March 16). Is social-skills training one "missing link"? *Education Week,* p. 45.

Leitman, R., & Binns, K. (1993). *The American teacher 1993: Violence in America's public schools.* New York: Louis Harris and Associates.

Leone, P. E., McLaughlin, M. J., & Meisel, S. M. (1992). School reform and adolescents with behavior disorders. *Focus on Exceptional Children, 25*(1), 1-15.

McGrew, K. S., Algozzine, B., Spiegel. A., Thurlow, M. L., & Ysseldyke, J. E. (1993). *The identification of people with disabilities in national data bases: A failure to communicate* (Technical Report No. 6). Minneapolis: University of Minnesota, National Center on Educational Outcomes.

McGrew, K. S., Spiegel, A., Thurlow, M. L., & Kim, D. (1994). *Matching information in national data collection programs to a model of school completion outcomes and indicators* (Technical Report No. 7). Minneapolis: University of Minnesota, National Center on Educational Outcomes.

McGrew, K. S., Thurlow, M. L., Shriner, J. G., & Spiegel, A. (1992). *Inclusion of students with disabilities in national and state data collection programs* (Technical Report No. 2). Minneapolis: University of Minnesota, National Center on Educational Outcomes.

National Education Goals Panel. (1993). *Statement on voluntary national education content standards* (Adopted November 15, 1993). Washington DC: Author.

OBE: What is the problem? (1994, June 30). *Minneapolis Star Tribune*, p. 16A.

O'Neil, J. (1992). Preparing for a changing workplace. *Educational Leadership* 49(6), 6-9.

Peacock Hill Working Group. (1991). Problem and promises in special education and related services for children and youth with emotional or behavioral disorders. *Behavioral Disorders, 16*(4), 299-313.

Porter, A. (1993). School delivery standards. *Educational Researcher, 22*(5), 24-30.

Rosenberg, M. S., Wilson, R., Maheady, L., & Sindelar, P. T. (1992). *Educating students with behavior disorders*. Boston: Allyn and Bacon.

Secretary's Commission on Achieving Necessary Skills. (1992). *Learning a living: A blueprint for high performance*. Washington, DC: U.S. Department of Labor.

Selden, R. (1992). National standards and testing. *State Board Connections–Issues in Brief, 12*(4), 1-5.

Shriner, J. G. (in press). Educational outcomes and standards for students with behavioral disorders: It's not just academics. *Education and Treatment of Children*.

Shriner, J. G., Bruininks, R. H., Deno, S. L., McGrew, K. S., Thurlow, M. L., & Ysseldyke, J. E. (1991). *State practices in the assessment of outcomes for students with disabilities* (Technical Report No. 1). Minneapolis: University of Minnesota, National Center on Educational Outcomes.

Shriner, J. G., & Thurlow, M. L. (1992). *State practices in the assessment of outcomes for students with disabilities: 1991*. Minneapolis: University of Minnesota, National Center on Educational Outcomes.

Shriner, J. G., Ysseldyke, J. E., Thurlow, M. L., & Honetschlager, D. (1994). "All" means "all"–Including students with disabilities. *Educational Leadership, 51*(6), 38-42.

Stemmer, P., Brown, W., & Smith, C. (1992). The employability skills portfolio. *Educational Leadership, 49*(6), 32-36.

Winget, P. (1994, April). Student outcomes should be consumer driven. *The Special Edge* (California State University), pp. 1,13.

Ysseldyke, J. E., Vanderwood, M., & Reschly, B. (1993). *Availability of data on school completion outcomes and indicators* (Technical Report No. 8). Minneapolis: University of Minnesota, National Center on Educational Outcomes.

Desired Results
of Second Chance Programs

Cheryl M. Lange
James E. Ysseldyke

University of Minnesota

SUMMARY. Are desired outcomes of schooling for students attending alternative schools similar to those for students attending typical high schools? Stakeholders representing students who attend alternative schools, teachers and directors from alternative schools, high school teachers, Directors of Special Education, and university teacher trainers participated in a consensus-building meeting. They reviewed and reached agreement on important indicators of educational outcomes for students attending alternative schools. Indicators were similar to those developed by personnel at the National Center on Educational Outcomes.

During the past decade, school choice has been implemented in several states. The opportunity for students to choose their school or

The development of this article was supported in part by a Cooperative Agreement (H023C00004) between the University of Minnesota and the U.S. Department of Education, Office of Special Education Programs. Points of view or opinions expressed in the article are not necessarily those of the department or offices within it.

Address correspondence to: Cheryl M. Lange, Open Enrollment Options for Students with Disabilities, 350 Elliott Hall, 75 East River Road, Minneapolis, MN 55455.

[Haworth co-indexing entry note]: "Desired Results of Second Chance Programs." Lange, Cheryl M., and James E. Ysseldyke. Co-published simultaneously in *Special Services in the Schools* (The Haworth Press, Inc.) Vol. 9, No. 2, 1994, pp. 155-171; and: *Educational Outcomes for Students with Disabilities* (ed: James E. Ysseldyke, and Martha L. Thurlow) The Haworth Press, Inc., 1994, pp. 155-171. Multiple copies of this article/chapter may be purchased from The Haworth Document Delivery Center [1-800-3-HAWORTH; 9:00 a.m. - 5:00 p.m. (EST)].

155

program has been embraced by many parents and educators. With school choice options gaining popularity, it is important to consider how programs will be evaluated and whether the outcomes will be different when students choose schools or programs that meet their unique needs.

There are many different forms of school choice options available, but second chance programs for students at risk of not completing school are of particular interest. Several states have adopted legislation that allows students who fit certain criteria (e.g., achievement discrepancies, expulsion, dropout, pregnant or custodial parent) the opportunity to transfer to another school district or to attend an alternative school or program (Cookson, 1994; Ysseldyke, Lange, & Delaney, 1992). While "alternative" has been used to describe many different types of schools or programs (Barr, Colston, Parrett, 1977; Nathan, 1976; Raywid, 1981), in this article we are interested in those programs that specifically address the needs of students at risk of not completing school.

There are several types of second chance option programs operating in many states. Though they may differ in their operation, they basically provide education for students who have had difficulty with the mainstream secondary school or traditional high school. This includes students with and without disabilities.

The programs are increasingly visible, but there is little documentation of their success in helping students meet the outcomes necessary for completing school. Many educators in alternative programs argue that their programs should be broadly evaluated, making sure that there is recognition of the unique population enrolled in the programs. These educators contend that the needs of students in their programs are extensive and often go beyond academics. Consequently, they believe that when evaluating the success of an alternative school or second chance program, students and programs must be judged on outcomes outside the academic domain. What those outcomes are for students attending second chance programs and how these compare to other school completion outcomes is of interest. As the population of students at-risk grows and as more and more students with disabilities access these programs, it is important to consider the outcomes for these students and their programs.

Minnesota has been a leader in the alternative school movement since the 1960s. There are over 135 alternative schools or Area Learning Centers (12 month schools with varied schedules and programs) in Minnesota. These programs have grown in number dramatically over the past five years. During the 1993-1994 school year, over 30,000 students chose to attend these programs. Many of these students are students with disabilities or special needs. Researchers at the Enrollment Options for Students with Disabilities Project at the University of Minnesota have been studying alternative schools and the role they play in the education of students with and without disabilities. Directors of alternative schools and Area Learning Centers completed surveys about student participation during the 1990-1991 school year. Directors indicated that approximately 19% of their students had disabilities or special needs. Over 50% were identified as being students with emotional behavioral disorders (Ysseldyke & Gorney, 1992).

Given the population of students served in alternative programs and their unique needs, do educators in the programs identify outcomes similar to those that have been broadly defined for the secondary school population? What outcomes do they believe to be most important to consider for the students participating in their programs? With programs that are meant to be alternative and out-of-the mainstream, how do these educators view the subject of outcomes for their students? These questions were put to a group of experts in the alternative school field in Minnesota. Using the model developed by the National Center on Educational Outcomes (NCEO), and the approach described in "A Guide . . . ," this volume, experts were asked to develop a list of indicators that could be used to evaluate students within alternative programs. In this paper, we delineate those found most important for students in these programs.

METHOD

Worksheets outlining the outcomes and indicators from the NCEO School Completion model (Ysseldyke, Thurlow, & Gilman, 1993) were distributed to 28 alternative school stakeholders. Included in the stakeholder group were students, alternative school teachers and directors, high school principals, high school teachers, directors of special education, department of education personnel, and university professors.

Stakeholders were asked to review the outcomes and indicators on the worksheet. The worksheet contained the outcomes and indicators for seven of the eight educational domains for school completion that had been developed by NCEO through a consensus building process involving educators from around the country. These domains include: (a) presence and participation, (b) physical health, (c) responsibility and independence, (d) citizenship and contribution, (e) academic and functional literacy, (f) personal and social adjustment, and (g) satisfaction. The eighth domain, accommodation and adaptation, was not included on the worksheet because this domain was not considered to be of primary importance for alternative schools. For each domain, stakeholders were asked to modify, delete, or add outcomes and indicators pertinent for students attending alternative schools or programs for students at risk of not completing school. A research assistant discussed the worksheets with the student respondents and noted their reactions. The other respondents returned the worksheets with their comments.

Twenty-five of the 28 stakeholders returned the worksheets. The responses were tallied and changes were made to a master indicator list. Following review of the completed worksheets, nine respondents were asked to attend a consensus building meeting designed to reach consensus on indicators most important for students in alternative schools. There was no differentiation between students with and without disabilities in the process since the original model was designed to be applicable to all students.

Multi-Attribute Consensus Building (MACB) (Vanderwood & Erickson, this volume; Vanderwood, Ysseldyke, & Thurlow, 1993), a process created by NCEO researchers using Multi-Attribute Utility Analysis (Lewis, Erickson, Johnson, & Bruininks, 1991), was used for group consensus building. Consensus was reached by asking participants to modify any indicator from the master list for which there was needed clarification. After discussion and agreement was reached on the wording of the indicators, participants rated the importance of each indicator from 0 to 100, for students attending alternative schools. Different indicators could have identical ratings. The only restriction was that one indicator had to be rated 100. With the assistance of computer technology, immediate feedback was available on changes to the wording of the indicators and on each participant's rating. The range of ratings and the mean for each indicator were displayed on a screen for all participants to view. Discussion followed each domain and participants were allowed to change their rating after the discussion period.

Participants were asked to rate the indicators in the context of student outcomes and not program outcomes. The wording of the outcomes and indicators was changed slightly from that in the NCEO model to account for this emphasis.

RESULTS

It is informative to look at the modified indicator lists for each domain, as well as the range, mean, and standard deviation for each indicator. It is also informative to note indicators that were removed by group consensus from the list. Some indicators had been added by the 28 stakeholders completing the worksheets, while others were part of the original indicator list from NCEO.

Presence and Participation

Participants and respondents noted that presence and participation indicators were very important for students attending alternative schools (see Table 1). However, the individualized nature of alternative schools influenced the interpretation of presence and participation. Because alternative school programs often include individualized learning plans, participants discussed the importance of students meeting the objectives in these plans as an indicator of success. This indicator was not on the original list of indicators from NCEO. However, group participants assigned it the highest rating for this domain, reflecting the delivery system in these schools and programs.

Participants added the indicator "the increase in quality of student efforts and achievements." There was consensus within the group that this was an important indicator of participation. Just being at school and completing work was not viewed as an index of

TABLE 1. Stakeholders' Ratings of Indicators for Presence and Participation

Indicator	Mean	SD	Min	Max
Shows progress on personal development plan.	96	9.4	70	100
Appropriately participates and communicates with students and staff.	94	8.3	80	100
Increase in quality of student efforts and achievements.	94	8.3	80	100
Rate of absenteeism during the school year (differentiated for reasons for suspension, medical/health condition, truancy and other reasons).	93	8.4	80	100
Number of credits/independent study units/requirements student completes.	89	13.4	60	100
Diploma/GED status.	88	12.9	60	100
Inactive status.	85	16.3	50	100
Elimiated/Modified Indicators:				
Actively engages in group discussions.				
GED status.				
Amount of independent study units satisfactorily completed.				
Communicates effectively with staff.				
Actively engages in group discussions.				

participation. The consensus group qualified and combined several indicators on classroom participation in the original model. They also discussed the importance of appropriate communication, since communication by itself was not a good indicator of participation.

Physical Health

Several indicators were added by the respondent and consensus group in the Physical Health domain (see Table 2). There was considerable concern about sleep habits, nutrition, and the reduction of at-risk behaviors. There was complete consensus on the importance of an indicator added by the consensus group: "if under

TABLE 2. Stakeholders' Ratings of Indicators for Physical Health

Indicator	Mean	SD	Min	Max
If under the influence of mood altering chemicals, does not engage in other high risk activities, i.e., driving, sexual practices, assault, etc.	100	0	100	100
Communicates an understanding of healthy sex practices.	99	3.3	90	100
Indicates use of protection against disease and unwanted pregnancy if sexually active.	99	3.3	90	100
Indicates reduction in the use of chemicals such as tobacco, drugs, alcohol, poisons, and inhalants.	95	10.0	70	100
Demonstrates knowledge of the dangers of chemical use such as use of tobacco, drugs, alcohol, poisons, and inhalants.	95	10.0	70	100
Indicates abstinence from chemical use.	91	11.4	70	100
Demonstrates awareness of basic health care needs.	89	12.7	60	100
Reduction of or abstinence from other high risk behaviors, i.e., carrying or possession of weapons.	87	16.4	60	100
Has healthy sleep habits.	86	17.6	50	100
Demonstrates knowledge of the health care system.	86	14.5	60	100
Demonstrates the appropriate use of over-the-counter drugs or prescription medicines.	86	14.1	60	100
Demonstrates knowledge of basic safety precautions and procedures.	85	11.5	70	100
Demonstrates healthy nutritional choices.	84	16.5	50	100
Participates in recreational and/or fitness activities.	83	16.0	50	100
Demonstrates knowledge of basic fitness needs.	81	15.6	50	100

Eliminated/Modified Indicators:

Demonstrates expected range of physical fitness.

the influence of mood altering chemicals, [student] does not engage in other high risk activities (i.e. driving, sexual practices, assault, etc.)."

Indicators addressing dangerous practices were added or modified at the meeting. Participants discussed the importance of abstinence or reduction of harmful activities and their relationship to success in other domain areas. Most of these indicators were rated high by the participant group. Only a single physical fitness indicator was deleted.

Responsibility and Independence

Both worksheet respondents and consensus group participants contributed changes to the indicators in the Responsibility and Independence domain (see Table 3). The participants pointed out that many of the students attending their schools were independent, but not necessarily exhibiting responsible behaviors. The most highly rated indicators in the final list reflect the group's emphasis on perseverance and follow-through on goals and activities.

Contribution and Citizenship

While several worksheet respondents added indicators for the domain of Contribution and Citizenship, the participants in the consensus group did not believe they belonged on a list of indicators for alternative school students. These are evident in Table 4. Individual indicators documenting illegal behavior or school disciplinary actions were included on the list of indicators with reservation. Though they were rated high, the group participants were concerned about the negative connotations of those indicators.

Indicators denoting knowledge of voting practices and actual voting were deleted, as were some indicators of community service. The group discussed the importance of these indicators but agreed they would not be important for students coming out of their programs.

Academic and Functional Literacy

There was nearly complete agreement on the indicators from the NCEO model in the Academic and Functional Literacy domain (see

TABLE 3. Stakeholders' Ratings for Indicators of Responsibility and Independence

Indicator	Mean	SD	Min	Max
Follows through on agreed upon school-related activities.	99	3.1	90	100
Perseveres toward goals.	97	6.7	80	100
Shows concern for others.	94	10.7	70	100
Sets and prioritizes goals.	94	9.6	70	100
Acts responsibly in a family or group.	92	13.7	60	100
Demonstrates the ability to manage time effectively.	90	9.1	75	100
Knows how to access community services, e.g., rehabilitation, counseling, employment, health care, etc.	87	11.3	70	100
Effectively advocates for him or herself.	86	9.8	70	100
Demonstrates the ability to complete transactions (shopping, banking, library) in the community.	84	10.7	70	100
Attends to own hygiene needs.	82	21.1	50	100
Likely to engage in life-long learning.	81	16.6	50	100
Manages personal budget.	79	13.4	50	100
Demonstrates the ability to get to and from a variety of destinations.	78	10.8	70	100
Takes care of own belongings.	72	18.1	50	90

Eliminated/Modified Indicators:

Demonstrates ability to read and follow city, state maps, and give accurate directions.

Table 5). Due to the high number of students in alternative programs who hold jobs outside school, work was added to environments where students should be capable of demonstrating academic and functional knowledge.

Personal and Social Adjustment

Participants deleted the indicator dealing with having friends and a social network from the NCEO model (see Table 6). After consid-

TABLE 4. Stakeholders' Ratings for Indicators of Contribution and Citizenship

Indicator	Mean	SD	Min	Max
Absence or reduced frequency of illegal behavior (e.g., shoplifting, vandalism, truancy, etc.).	96	7.3	80	100
Makes a positive contribution to the classroom environment.	96	8.8	75	100
Demonstrates responsibility for the environment.	94	7.3	80	100
Absence or reduced frequency of suspension or disciplinary actions.	92	9.9	75	100
Demonstrates knowledge of the democratic process.	84	17.4	60	100
Understands the significance of community service or is involved in community service.	81	15.5	60	100

Eliminated/Modified Indicators:

Absence or reduced frequency of involvement with the criminal justice system.

Knows the procedures necessary to register and vote.

Is registered to vote at age 18.

Is familiar with the candidates and issues during election campaigns.

Volunteers time to school, civic, community, or non-profit activities.

Supports a charity organization either emotionally or financially.

erable discussion, consensus could not be reached and the participants thought the indicator should not be included because there were too many intervening variables. While having friends, and a social network is an indicator of social and personal adjustment, there was concern that the type of friends or social network can work against positive adjustment. It was suggested that they could qualify the type of friendships; but, participants did not want to place a value on friendships. Instead, they decided to eliminate the entire indicator.

The Personal and Social Adjustment domain was considered to be very important for many of the respondents and participants. On

TABLE 5. Stakeholders' Ratings of Indicators for Academic and Functional Literacy

Indicator	Mean	SD	Min	Max
Effectively uses communication skills.	100	0	100	100
Demonstrates problem solving and critical thinking skills.	100	0	100	100
Demonstrates competence in other skills necessary to function in current home, school, work and community environments.	100	0	100	100
Demonstrates competence in other skills necessary to function in next environments.	100	0	100	100
Demonstrates competence in math necessary to function in next environments.	99	3.1	90	100
Demonstrates competence in reading necessary to function in next environments.	99	3.1	90	100
Demonstrates competence in writing necessary to function in next environments.	99	3.1	90	100
Demonstrates competence in math necessary to function in current home, school, work, and community environments.	98	6.3	80	100
Demonstrates competence in reading necessary to function in current home, school, work, and community environments.	98	6.3	80	100
Demonstrates competence in writing necessary to function in current home, school, work, and community environments.	98	6.3	80	100
Applies technology to enhance functioning in home, school, work, and community environments.	98	6.3	80	100
Demonstrates competence in using technology to function in next environments.	97	6.7	80	100

Eliminated/Modified Indicators:

Participates in work experience/vocational training program.

TABLE 6. Stakeholders' Ratings of Indicators for Personal and Social Adjustment

Indicator	Mean	SD	Min	Max
Recognizes and respects similarities and differences between self and others.	97	4.7	90	100
Demonstrates knowledge of appropriate boundaries in relationships.	97	5.3	85	100
Expresses feelings and needs in socially acceptable ways.	97	6.7	80	100
Deals appropriately with personal challenges, frustrations, and stressors.	96	5.7	85	100
Perceives him or herself as worthwhile and competent.	96	6.9	80	100
Demonstrates cultural sensitivity through behavior, language, and ability to educate others.	96	6.9	80	100
Accepts responsibility for their own behavior and its consequences.	96	8.1	75	100
Demonstrates skill in managing interpersonal conflict.	94	6.9	80	100
Shows respect for differing opinions.	91	12.0	60	100
Engages in productive group work in home, school, or community settings.	86	14.2	50	100
Shows optimism about his or her future.	79	13.4	50	100
Relates appropriately to authority.	77	27.9	0	90
Behavior reflects an appropriate degree of self-control.	73	1.1	0	100

Eliminated/Modified Indicators:

Deals appropriately with frustration and unfavorable events.

Demonstrates ability to educate others to recognize their need to be more accepting of cultural differences.

Has friends and is part of a social network.

Demonstrates skill in interacting and in making decisions in social situations, including during interpersonal conflict.

several occasions, participants discussed how positive indicators in this domain were necessary prerequisites to academic and functional literacy. They expressed the importance they place on these indicators within their programs (see Table 7).

Satisfaction

Since this group was using the NCEO model to determine indicators at the student level and not at a program accountability level, there was some confusion about the role of parents and community in this domain. To eliminate confusion, participants were asked to concentrate on indicators of student satisfaction. Many participants voiced concern over parent and community satisfaction, but the group decided that including parent and community indicators was not necessary for understanding student satisfaction.

Worksheet respondents added an indicator for the satisfaction

TABLE 7. Stakeholders' Ratings of Indicators for Satisfaction

Indicator	Mean	SD	Min	Max
Student's satisfaction with level of achievement.	99	3.5	90	100
Student's satisfaction with alternative program experience.	96	10.5	70	100
Student's satisfaction with what is being provided in school.	93	13.8	60	100
Intends to pursue further learning experiences.	88	16.4	50	100
Parent's/guardian's perception of student's satisfaction with the alternative program experience.	86	12.1	40	100
Parent's guardian's satisfaction with alternative program experience.	84	14.3	60	100

Eliminated/Modified Indicators:

Student's satisfaction with progress toward achieving educational outcomes.

Parent's satisfaction with what is being provided in school.

Parent's satisfaction with progress toward achieving educational outcomes.

Community's satisfaction with the extent to which student is prepared to live in society.

domain that involved future learning experiences. The consensus participants agreed that it would be a good indicator of satisfaction.

Since many of the students' parents are not actively involved in the students' educational programs, or the students are living independently, there was discussion about the importance of parent satisfaction. The group decided to add an indicator involving parents' perceptions of student satisfaction and keep one indicator denoting parental satisfaction with their child's alternative school experience.

DISCUSSION

Discussions with educators in alternative programs during the past year have brought attention to the need to evaluate students and programs over a range of outcomes and indicators. Researchers were often reminded that when doing research on alternative programs and students, it is important to include all areas of development and curriculum that influence academic and functional success. Educators voiced concern that only those outcomes directly associated with academic success would be used for student or program evaluation.

The broad array of domains, outcomes, and indicators presented in the NCEO model pleased respondents. There was agreement that all of these areas were important for students in alternative schools. There also was agreement by consensus participants that attainment of indicators in some domains was essential before success could be gauged in the academic areas.

Participants and worksheet respondents noted the important role certain domain areas play in their programs. For example, the interpretation of presence and participation is crucial to understanding the success of the student in an alternative program. Often, students in these programs come and go from the programs several times during the school year. However, they may still be considered participants in learning if they continue to work toward reaching the goals on their individual learning plans.

Consensus group participants were particularly concerned about physical health indicators. They discussed the high risk behavior of their students. Demonstrating knowledge of the dangers of chemical substance use and unprotected sexual practices were considered important indicators of understanding the importance of physical health issues. However, participants stressed that abstinence from and reduction of high risk behaviors were also essential indicators to include in this domain. Participants discussed the indicators in this domain in relationship to student academic success. Substance abuse and other high risk behaviors can often be the barrier to academic success. The importance of dealing with behaviors that create barriers was emphasized by group participants.

There was lively group discussion when reviewing the responsibility and independence goals for alternative school students. Many participants pointed out that some of their students lived independently or were independent from the control of their parents or guardians. Therefore, evaluating independence was discussed within a unique context. Many of the students were exhibiting independent behaviors by virtue of their living arrangements. However, behaviors showing responsibility and independence within the school setting were not always in congruence with the independent behavior exhibited in their day-to-day living. With this noted by several participants, the group decided to limit indicators to those most directly observed in the school setting. Again, discussants noted the importance of setting goals, prioritizing them, and following through on activities as behaviors related to academic success.

As was the case with the other domains, personal and social adjustment indicators were discussed in relationship to academic success. Little could be accomplished academically for some students if they were not able to demonstrate personal and social adjustment, responsibility, an understanding of physical health issues, or act appropriately, etc.

These educators strongly advocated evaluating students individually with emphasis on the goals they had set and needed to accomplish before moving to the next step in their school program. For some students this may mean strong emphasis on reaching outcomes in the areas of physical health and for others meeting outcomes in academic literacy. There was consensus that all the needs of the individual student had to be considered and evaluated without placing importance on only one domain area. Often, success in one domain would be the key to success in another domain. The challenge for educators was to help the students identify goals and reach them so they could eventually be successful in each of the areas. This did not mean, however, that indicators in domain areas were mutually exclusive. Student goals reflected the array of domains as did the indicators of success. Again, participants stressed the importance of all areas and the importance of evaluation in all areas, without total success being gauged within those traditionally labeled academic.

Individuals and their needs were emphasized by both the participants and worksheet respondents. Students who discussed the worksheets also saw the importance of the individual, but from a perspective that included rejection of many of the indicators in areas that educators in alternative programs agreed were important. These included the physical health and social and personal adjustment domains. It was interesting to receive feedback from these students and to document the differences in importance placed on these domains.

The list of indicators presented by the consensus group is altered some from that of the stakeholders who developed this model for the NCEO. Most indicators, however, remain the same. The direction this group gave to the outcomes discussion centers on individual needs and individual goals. They are eager for evaluation of their students and programs; but, are anxious about how that will be accomplished if those evaluating do not consider the enormous importance of indicators in domains not traditionally measured. The clientele and their needs dictate that outcomes be considered over many domains to fairly evaluate the students and their programs.

Special services staff can benefit from the information provided by experts in the field of alternative education. More and more students with disabilities are accessing alternative schools. As these schools become more prevalent special educators often make decisions or recommendations about the possibility of alternative schools for particular students. Issues relating to special education services must also be addressed when students with disabilities enroll in alternative schools or programs. Understanding the outcomes and indicators considered important by the educators in these settings can help special services staff with decision making about students and special services within these settings.

REFERENCES

Barr, R. D., Colston, B., & Parrett, W. H. (1977). The effectiveness of alternative public schools. *Viewpoints, 53*(4), 1-30.

Cookson, P. W. Jr. (1994). *School choice: The struggle for the soul of American education.* New Haven: Yale University Press.

Gorney, D. J., & Ysseldyke, J. E. (1993). Students with disabilities use of various options to access alternative schools and Area Learning Centers. *Special Services in the Schools, 7*(1), 125-143.

Lewis, D. R., Erickson, R. N., Johnson, D. R., & Bruininks, R. H. (1991). *Using multi-attribute utility evaluation techniques in special education.* Unpublished manuscript, University of Minnesota, Institute on Community Integration, Minneapolis.

Nathan, J. (1976). Let us be extremely frank: A concise history of public alternative schools. *New Schools Exchange Newsletter, 132,* 4-13.

Raywid, M. A. (1981). The first decade of public school alternatives. *Phi Delta Kappan, 62*(8), 551-573.

Vanderwood, M., Ysseldyke, J., & Thurlow, M. (1993). *Consensus building: A process for selecting educational outcomes and indicators.* Minneapolis: University of Minnesota, National Center on Educational Outcomes.

Ysseldyke, J. E., & Gorney, D. J. (1992). *Students with disabilities use of various options to access alternative schools and Area Learning Centers.* Research Report No. 3, Enrollment Options for Students with Disabilities Project. Minneapolis, MN: University of Minnesota.

Ysseldyke, J. E., Lange, C. M., & Delaney, T. J. (1992). *School choice programs in the fifty states.* Research Report No. 7, Enrollment Options for Students with Disabilities Project. Minneapolis, MN: University of Minnesota.

Ysseldyke, J. E., Thurlow, M. L., & Gilman, C. J. (1993). *Educational outcomes and indicators for students completing school.* Minneapolis: University of Minnesota, National Center on Educational Outcomes.

Stakeholder Reactions to Developing a Model for Early Childhood

Cheri J. Gilman

St. Cloud State University

SUMMARY. This paper examines reactions to the NCEO early childhood outcomes models by three types of stakeholder groups (administrators/policy makers, early interventionists/teachers, and parents). Individuals within these groups represent either a general early childhood perspective or an early childhood special education perspective. Several issues that emerged are presented, and unresolved issues are discussed.

Local, state and national policymakers have increasingly focused on specific indicators that could be used to measure progress in enhancing important developmental and educational outcomes for children and youth. The emphasis of recent efforts has been primarily on defining specific outcomes and indicators, and the possible measures that are appropriate sources of data. Less emphasis has been placed on the *process* of selecting important outcomes and indicators. This paper examines issues surrounding the use of a conceptual model of educational outcomes and indicators developed by the National Center on Educational Outcomes (NCEO) at

Address correspondence to: Cheri J. Gilman, Child and Family Studies, Education Building B 109, SCSU, 720 Fourth Avenue South, St. Cloud, MN 56301-4498.

[Haworth co-indexing entry note]: "Stakeholder Reactions to Developing a Model for Early Childhood." Gilman, Cheri J. Co-published simultaneously in *Special Services in the Schools* (The Haworth Press, Inc.) Vol. 9, No. 2, 1994, pp. 173-180; and: *Educational Outcomes for Students with Disabilities* (ed: James E. Ysseldyke, and Martha L. Thurlow) The Haworth Press, Inc., 1994, pp. 173-180. Multiple copies of this article/chapter may be purchased from The Haworth Document Delivery Center [1-800-3-HAWORTH; 9:00 a.m. - 5:00 p.m. (EST)].

the University of Minnesota (see Gilman, Thurlow, & Ysseldyke, 1992; NCEO, 1992; Ysseldyke et al., 1991; Ysseldyke et al., 1992). The focus on the process of selecting those important outcomes and indicators is reflected in the systematic involvement of multiple stakeholders with potentially diverse perspectives in consensus building procedures. To suggest there is "a definitive list" of important outcomes in any area is to put oneself out on a limb. It is crucial that we keep in mind that the development of outcomes is an ongoing process; no single listing will capture the complexities of what are important outcomes for all individuals in the context of their own families and communities. It is also crucial that we continue to chart a course that keeps practitioners, administrators, policymakers and parents attending to important outcomes for our children and youth (with and without disabilities). Charting a clear course is the first step to reaching the destination.

The current educational climate is one of increasing participation of various stakeholders in decision making and of moving toward greater inclusion of students with disabilities in regular education initiatives. The importance assigned to specific outcomes should influence policy and practice regarding measurement and accountability.

THE HISTORICAL CONTEXT

Recent legislation has increased our focus on the welfare of our nation's youngest and most vulnerable citizens, that is, children in the "early childhood" infant and preschool years. P.L. 99-457, for example, extended states' accountability for young children with disabilities downward to age three. In addition, it emphasized a family-focused approach to systematically involve parents in the process of defining goals for children with disabilities beginning from birth. The Bank Street survey (Marx & Seligson, 1988) was an initial attempt to gather national information on early childhood programs. In attempting to build a uniform data base across states and program areas, these researchers concluded that there was a need to develop a national data base for pre-kindergarten services. Only after a framework of important educational outcomes and indicators of those outcomes is established, however, can the process move forward to any set of coherent measurement standards. With the increasing emphasis on reform in our educational system, particularly the establishment of national goals, efforts in this area of policy research provide an important opportunity to begin to link outcomes and indicators to educational goals that have been expressed in legislation and policy.

THE CONCEPTUAL FRAMEWORK OF OUTCOMES

As a result of various working papers and consensus meetings of stakeholders representing policymakers, researchers, educators and parents of children with and without disabilities, NCEO developed its framework of domains, outcomes and indicators (see "What Results . . . ," this volume). While the model has a "finished" look about it, again it is important to view it as under development. The eight domains should be useful in defining the parameters within which outcomes and indicators of those outcomes can be developed and validated. But, at what point do we limit debate on changing the parameters of outcome domains and labels for those domains? This issue was debated up front and is reflected in a series of working papers. It was only at the early childhood level that any substantive change was made to the model. The specification of "family involvement/accommodation and adaptation" in the early childhood age groups broadened the perspective beyond holding children accountable for outcomes to providing families and communities with the support that is needed to help children reach those outcomes.

It appears that any real debate about the early childhood model generally centers around the indicators. Coming to consensus about broad domains or fairly broad outcomes that are important is less of an issue than the indicators we choose to reflect achievement or mastery of those outcomes. "Demonstrating age-appropriate independence" (an outcome) is something that is likely to get fairly high agreement as to its importance. The possible indicators of such an outcome may be contested, however, depending on your developmental perspective of what "age-appropriate" might mean and what cultural values you hold about independence. Indicators of this outcome such as, "easy separation from parents/guardians in familiar and comfortable situations" and "remaining occupied without continuous adult involvement" may not get the same level of support within and across various stakeholder groups. The approximately 20 outcomes and 60 indicators of those outcomes in the conceptual framework of outcomes and indicators developed through NCEO's consensus process for early childhood (that is, at a point in a continuum around age 3) does not reflect a definitive list of all possible outcomes and indicators. The framework does provide, however, a starting point from which debate can begin about what it is we value on a local, state or national level in terms of important outcomes for young children. The process itself, of suggesting indicators of outcomes in an open forum where they can be assigned relative weights and debated, is helpful in moving us toward consensus. Rather than simply collecting data and measuring what is easy to measure, shouldn't we be deciding what it is we value and finding a way to determine how we can measure our progress?

BETWEEN AND WITHIN STAKEHOLDER BOUNDARIES

If our national education goals are intended to mean "all" children, then it is important that we begin with such a premise at the early childhood level with a model of outcomes and indicators that is intended to be inclusive of all children, but that we also gain greater understanding of how different stakeholders value outcomes for young children. Simply saying we want a model to "include all children" may not make it so. Two of the domains in NCEO's model, in particular, have a "special education" ring to them. Who is likely to be concerned with children and youth being "present and participating" and having "accommodations and adaptations" to meet outcomes in all domains? These are not typically the focus of regular educators, but are what special educators view as important opportunities for children and youth with special needs. How, then, will a group of stakeholders that only represents the regular education perspective value these domains and their corresponding outcomes and indicators?

In a recent study designed to compare the perspectives of six classes of stakeholder groups in Minnesota, including administrators/policy makers, early interventionists/teachers, and parents of young children representing either early childhood or early childhood special education perspectives (Gilman, 1994), several issues emerged that are important to consider. These are illustrated by focusing on one domain and the outcomes and indicators within that domain.

1. The mean ratings of these six stakeholder subgroups for the broad domain "presence and participation" showed little variation. All were between 82 and 90 (on a scale of 0-100). In consensus process "rules" for deciding whether something is an important item to keep in the model, it would appear, as a domain, to be valued and thus retained by all. This finding supports the earlier statement that the level of debate does not center around broad outcome domains.

2. The mean ratings for outcomes that reflected either "presence" or "participation" were lower than the ratings for the domain as a whole. They ranged from 68-80. In all comparisons between regular and special education respondents, the level of support for these two outcomes was higher from the special education respondents. In this sample then, it appears that in this domain with a "special education" ring to it, there is indeed more support from the special education community for these particular outcomes. If such differences were to hold and be significant across large samples, we need to ask ourselves what this means for policy and practice in the context of inclusion of children with disabilities in mainstream settings.

3. The variation in the ratings of the eight indicators of presence and participation was evident across the six subgroups of stakeholders and across the eight indicators. This lends support to the earlier argument about where the level of debate lies. The mean rage in ratings was from 44-93. Five of the eight indicators received enough support (i.e., ratings of 75 and above by all stakeholder subgroups) to be retained by this sample of respondents.

4. Indicators that did not receive support from the six stakeholder subgroups were all items that had wording that could be described as "negative" indicators rather than "positive" indicators. The instructions given to the respondents stated that negatively worded items did not mean you endorsed the item, per se, but valued collecting information on that particular indicator. "Absenteeism from daycare, preschool or other early childhood programs," for example, was given lower ratings by all respondent groups. An item so worded raises a debate as to whether the respondents indeed did not

care about absenteeism rates or they did not want to rate absenteeism high because they thought not being absent was important. In developing NCEO's conceptual model of outcomes and indicators, those who provided reactions to the early working papers raised the issue of negatively worded indicators. It appears the concerns of those who emphasized that all indicators should be worded in a positive manner were warranted. In building consensus around indicators, it is important to know whether respondents are interpreting the item in the same manner. Dialogue during the process, of course, could provide such clarification, but items needing little or no clarification would be preferred. Without that clarification, does the 10-point mean difference in this sample between parents of typically developing young children and children with special needs mean that parents of typically developing children are less concerned about absenteeism? Does it mean that parents of children with special needs have a heightened awareness due to their children's more frequent medical needs of the importance of not being absent? The lack of clarity in how such indicators might have been interpreted by the respondents makes these inferences impossible.

5. The eight indicators that were in this domain were in the model because they were retained by the consensus process that involved representatives across broad stakeholder groups. The interaction/dialog that was possible during the consensus process involving stakeholders with differing perspectives allowed for clarification and changing support that was not possible in a survey format where the ratings of stakeholders within specific subgroups were compared. The results, however, of this sample, in which five indicators were retained lends support to the use of those indicators by the subsample that rated them. Not all of the indicators will be important within the context of various localities/programs. It is a strength of such a model to permit different valuing of what is important to use as indicators of success for various outcomes.

6. Often the focus has been on isolated outcomes or indicators. In using the MAU consensus process (see Vanderwood & Erickson, this volume), respondents rated the value of outcome domains, outcomes and indicators. In so doing, this process goes beyond isolated items. The interaction of the overall ratings of the broad outcome domains with outcomes and indicators provides a three-tiered look.

A highly valued indicator, for example, in a domain and/or outcome that is not highly valued will have less importance than an equally valued indicator in a more highly valued domain and/or outcome. Use of such information in policy and program decisions may help ensure that we are collecting the kind of information in the kind of areas that we value. With increasing emphasis on accountability and the need to protect the public's investment in early education, it is important to give direction to programs in terms of the outcomes that are valued by stakeholders.

UNRESOLVED ISSUES

While conceptual models are extremely important to researchers and policymakers to facilitate communication, there is some frustration in the constraints such models put upon those involved in a consensus process. With respect to the early childhood consensus meetings that were convened to refine the model at ages 3 and 6, the question of whether domains intended to span ages from preschool through postschool were indeed the "ideal" domains for early childhood was an issue. Starting from scratch was viewed as an attractive alternative by participants in the midst of trying to "fit" their perspectives within an existing model. We need to question, however, how many times we can start the process from scratch. Consistency across a model can be viewed as an advantageous framework as long as there is enough flexibility to modify and amend it to suit particular age-related or locality needs.

A final issue is the expressed discomfort of many parents involved in the consensus process of placing relative weights to outcomes and indicators. Both in consensus meetings and in the follow-up survey format, parents seem to struggle with having to consider and rate the relative merits of specific items. How we prepare parents for and include them in our consensus processes warrants some consideration. What we need to be cautious about is that the discomfort in valuing items (especially those that are unclear or jargon-laden) does not get played out in diminished participation. There are differences in perspectives and having each of them represented in the process is critical for the effort to be a meaningful one. Including parents as partners in educational planning and decision making is viewed as important but is often not carried out effectively. The use of the multiattribute consensus process in this study may be one means by which such partnerships can be facilitated. Professionals are increasingly working toward facilitating meaningful parent input into the development of specific learning outcomes for their own children. Parent input can be facilitated on a broader policy level when parents share in the process with professionals in specifying the valued outcome areas, outcomes and related indicators of outcomes for early childhood in general.

CONCLUSION

Whenever administrators or policymakers shift the focus to examining outcomes and indicators at the early childhood level or beyond, input from all stakeholders is crucial. The NCEO conceptual model may be useful as a framework. Using specific domains, outcomes, and indicators, and applying a consensus-building approach seems to provide the breadth and flexibility required to create a product that reflects what is valued by the participating stakeholders.

REFERENCES

Gilman, C. J., Thurlow, M. L., & Ysseldyke, J. E. (1992). *Responses to Working Paper 1: Conceptual model of educational outcomes for children and youth with disabilities* (Synthesis Report 3). Minneapolis, MN: National Center on Educational Outcomes, University of Minnesota.

Gilman, C. J. (1994). Consensual validation of early childhood outcomes and indicators. Unpublished manuscript.

Marx, F. & Seligson, M. (1988). *The public school early childhood study: The state survey.* New York: Bank Street College of Education.

NCEO. (1992). *State special education outcomes 1991.* Minneapolis, MN: National Center on Educational Outcomes, University of Minnesota.

Ysseldyke, J. E., Thurlow, M. L., Bruininks, R. H., Deno, S. L., McGrew, K. S., & Shriner, J. G. (1991). *A conceptual model of educational outcomes for children and youth with disabilities.* (Working Paper 1). Minneapolis, MN: National Center on Educational Outcomes, University of Minnesota.

Ysseldyke, J. E., Thurlow, M. L., Bruininks, R. H., Gilman, C. J., Deno, S. L., McGrew, K. S., & Shriner, J.G. (1992). *An evolving conceptual model of educational outcomes for children and youth with disabilities* (Working Paper 2). Minneapolis, MN: National Center on Educational Outcomes, University of Minnesota.

Beyond Traditional Standards:
A Personal Perspective

Nancy Verderber

Special School District
St. Louis, Missouri

SUMMARY. The needs of students with disabilities are often forgotten in discussions of educational outcomes and standards. It is important to consider the perspective of people with disabilities when thinking about outcomes. Recognition of this perspective implies that school personnel, with the leadership of special services personnel, need to identify the ways (sometimes through modifications and adaptations) in which students can achieve outcomes.

The establishment of educational outcomes for children with disabilities is essentially about creating a vision and philosophy which supports each child's natural abilities. Appropriate early childhood educational supports will ensure successful outcomes for students with disabilities. I well recall being a child with a physical disability label that told the world, and myself, that "you are different." Preschool children are made aware of expectations early on, such as tying shoes, dressing, skipping, running, etc. These, in turn, become standards by which the educational system determines appropriate outcomes. Unfortunately the system has been remiss in recognizing the need to adapt and modify outcomes for students with disabilities.

Address correspondence to: Nancy Verderber, Special School District, 12110 Clayton Road, St. Louis, MO 63131.

[Haworth co-indexing entry note]: "Beyond Traditional Standards: A Personal Perspective." Verderber, Nancy. Co-published simultaneously in *Special Services in the Schools* (The Haworth Press, Inc.) Vol. 9, No. 2, 1994, pp. 181-184; and: *Educational Outcomes for Students with Disabilities* (ed: James E. Ysseldyke, and Martha L. Thurlow) The Haworth Press, Inc., 1994, pp. 181-184. Multiple copies of this article/chapter may be purchased from The Haworth Document Delivery Center [1-800-3-HAWORTH; 9:00 a.m. - 5:00 p.m. (EST)].

This does not mean that they are not expected to succeed . . . it means that it is the responsibility of the educators and parents to identify how a student can achieve an outcome, possibly in a different way.

If the typical standards had been held for me, I would still be in pre-school! Due to the wonderful notion of common sense, utilized by my teachers and family, I escaped the punishment of strict standards for educational outcomes. It sure didn't take me long to figure out that I wasn't able to tie my shoes or color in between the lines. For some of my early professionals the concept of finding a different way to accomplish outcomes, i.e., writing, was very foreign to them. Some school personnel and other professionals could not move past the mentality that they had to fix me before I could move on. Unfortunately, as a school administrator I find that this is often still the case.

I read an article several years ago entitled "Dismantling the Poster Child Image" (Denti, 1992) which eloquently points out the decades of attitudinal disservice to youngsters with disabilities. Society tends to perpetuate the feelings of pity for children with disabilities and sorrow for their families. Early childhood educational outcomes for children with disabilities must place the child on an equal playing field with all children. That might come in the form of adaptation or modification in the curriculum, environment and, more importantly, attitudes of teachers, parents and administrators.

Very often, school officials and parents of children with disabilities ask me, "What did your parents do that made you so self-sufficient?" I always smile and think to myself that they just treated me like their six other children. I had fun, got into trouble and received lots of love (and continue to do so!)!

When I really think about it, it's amazing that my parents were able to raise me like my siblings because society tried its best to relay messages to treat me differently and "special."

My first education in self-advocacy occurred at the age of four. I recall loving to go uptown to shop with my mother, sisters and brothers. My hometown, Lincoln, Illinois, is relatively small. Most everyone knows each other. The well-meaning, but patronizing, sales clerks would always ask my mother, "What's her name, how old is she?" but never look at me. I would occasionally get the proverbial head pat!

I'm sure they felt sorry for me, seeing me slouched in a stroller supported by pillows and involuntarily moving my arms because of my cerebral palsy. Nevertheless, my mother and I devised a plan to educate these people without their knowledge (little did we know that this would go on forever!). My mother would simply turn away when asked my name or age. From my stroller I would say as loudly as possible, "Nancy. I'm four years old!" (This was the best form of speech therapy.)

This scenario has been played out over and over throughout my life. My parents must have been frustrated at times, but they continued with humor and forthrightness. I'm sure glad they let me know when people spoke about me out of ignorance when I wasn't present instead of hiding it from me. One day my mother brought groceries to the car and had a smile on her face. She informed me, at the age of ten, that the overly friendly checkout lady was wanting to know when "that girl" of hers was going to die! In our laughter, we were also angry.

My dad, being silent and strong, continued to be a big asset in my accidental mainstreaming (before P.L. 94-142). Instead of working a 9 to 5 job with security, he utilized his wonderful talents as a self-employed carpenter and tile contractor. He took me to and from school, never making it the burden that society may have viewed it as, but just a part of life.

Like all kids, I wanted a bike but my parents were unable to adapt one. Instead, they compensated with a go-cart with pedals. This was probably the best form of physical therapy that I could have had.

The stories could go on forever. Therefore, I want to share some tips that worked for my educational benefit:

1. Have age-appropriate expectations which are flexible with modifications and/or adaptations.
2. Give students with disabilities classroom responsibilities. Also provide choices (verbal or nonverbal).
3. Praise actions appropriately. (Don't overdo it!)
4. Recognize the child's abilities, gifts and talents rather than focusing on the attributes of the child's disability. After all, would you want everyone to know about your bowel, bladder and feeding habits?
5. Children with disabilities aren't always "angels" or "special." They can be manipulative, aggravating little monsters,

just like all children! Don't be afraid to appropriately reprimand a child with disabilities when needed, like any child.
6. Don't use baby talk when addressing students–they are no longer babies. Speak in a normal tone of voice.
7. Definitely have a sense of humor.
8. Incorporate dignity and self-respect. (It's O.K. to be disabled.) As the Americans with Disabilities Act states, "Being disabled is part of the human experience."
9. Introduce the child to a person with a similar disability who has a positive attitude. This can be one of the greatest role models that the child will ever have!!
10. Enjoy students of all abilities–they grow fast. Keep your hopes and dreams alive for their future, but be flexible. No one knows the future, no one is perfect.

Successful inclusion of early childhood students with disabilities into our educational system is a matter of attitude and knowledge of state-of-the-art practices. Many teachers express to me that they are not sure if they know how to include. I always respond that they do . . . by giving the example of family gatherings. At Thanksgiving, many families come together with a wide range of people, personalities and ages. The bottom line is to make them feel welcome, valued and loved.

The same bottom line is true for inclusion in the classroom. As the host (or teacher) one must find how activities throughout the day can be offered so that everyone benefits. Scrabble is a popular game on Thanksgiving in my household. We have six year olds to a 91 year old playing. Last Thanksgiving it dawned on me how much we continuously adjust to make inclusion of all players work, with the youngest spelling words like "cat" or "dog" and the oldest requiring much patience.

Classroom inclusion is much like our Scrabble game. I truly believe we will successfully have accomplished school inclusion when we don't have to label it, but just call it "going to school" like I did back in the 60s.

REFERENCE

Denti, L. (1989, December). Dismantling the poster child image. *Mainstream.*

Parental Perspectives
on Educational Outcomes

Ann P. Turnbull

Beach Center on Families and Disability
University of Kansas

Janet R. Vohs

Federation for Children with Special Needs
Boston, Massachusetts

SUMMARY. The language of the NCEO early childhood model illustrates the risks in developing a system of outcomes and indicators. Though the early childhood model clearly attempts to be inclusive, some of its assumptions and its emphasis upon normal development and age appropriateness work contrary to this intention. This article emphasizes including parents in the process of developing a model for early childhood education, and recommends that we look not only at the support that parents provide to their children for reaching educational outcomes, but also the support received by the parents. A final recommendation, proposed in this article, addresses the composition of the stakeholders involved in developing a model of outcomes and indicators.

We would like to address four major issues including: (a) the stated assumptions that the outcomes should address the needs of all

---

Address correspondence to: Ann P. Turnbull, the Beach Center on Families and Disabilities, University of Kansas, 3111 Haworth Hall, Lawrence, KS 66045.

[Haworth co-indexing entry note]: "Parental Perspectives on Educational Outcomes." Turnbull, Ann P., and Janet R. Vohs. Co-published simultaneously in *Special Services in the Schools* (The Haworth Press, Inc.) Vol. 9, No. 2, 1994, pp. 185-191; and: *Educational Outcomes for Students with Disabilities* (ed: James E. Ysseldyke, and Martha L. Thurlow) The Haworth Press, Inc., 1994, pp. 185-191. Multiple copies of this article/chapter may be purchased from The Haworth Document Delivery Center [1-800-3-HAWORTH; 9:00 a.m. - 5:00 p.m. (EST)].

students, (b) the standards of normality and age-appropriateness, (c) the outcomes and indicators that address family involvement, and (d) the composition of stakeholder groups.

ASSUMPTIONS CONCERNING ALL CHILDREN

The NCEO model made the first assumption that outcomes should apply to *all* students. We believe that an inclusive approach and unitary thinking is exactly on target. The second NCEO assumption, however, appears to contradict the first one: "Indicators of outcomes for students receiving special education services should be related, conceptually and statistically, to those identified for students without disabilities." If there is an assumption for a unitary system, it appears incongruent to then address two categories of outcomes. The second assumption makes us uncomfortable in its impression that developing a unitary system means that special education needs to *conform* to general education. To continue our thinking toward creating a unitary system, true reform implies something new, not yet expressed in terms such as "general" or "special" education but built upon strengths from both arenas.

We have some recommendations for changes in the wording of the outcomes based on an inclusive philosophy. In the Presence and Participation Domain, there is an outcome: "Is present in group activities." An alternative would be "Demonstrates membership in the school community," since such an outcome would be possible for alternative ways of participating–from a hospital bed, via computer, or just by showing up. In the Responsibility and Independence Domain, emphasis might be given to initiative and interdependence rather than independence. Finally, within the Contribution and Citizenship Domain, we take exception to the selection of outcomes related only to "compliance" and "acceptance." Alternative outcomes more clearly aligned with the Domains of Contribution and Citizenship and expressing stronger themes of belonging and initiative might be:

- Demonstrates awareness/appreciation of own gifts
- Demonstrates appreciation of others' gifts
- Demonstrates confidence in self

- Demonstrates ability to include others
- Demonstrates belonging/membership in the school community.

Our major point is that the philosophy of inclusion—where all students belong—does not consistently pervade these outcomes and indicators. The Domain of Citizenship certainly seems a most logical context in which to raise issues related to building community.

EMPHASIS ON NORMAL DEVELOPMENT AND AGE APPROPRIATENESS

Three types of criteria operate across domains: (a) normal development (Physical Health Domain); (b) age-appropriateness (Responsibility and Independence Domain; Contribution and Citizenship Domain); and (c) general descriptors of competence without a normal developmental or age-appropriate expectation (Academic and Functional Literacy Domain; Presence and Participation Domain; and Personal and Social Adjustment Domains). We have grave concerns about the emphasis on normal development and age-appropriateness. For example, in the Physical Health Domain, an outcome is "Demonstrates normal physical development." The fact that such terminology could appear here attests to the power of unstated norms that currently guide educational thinking and to the need to be rigorous in selecting a vocabulary that is appropriate to a reformed unitary system. The current understanding of normality is very narrow, and disability is not generally considered normal. Thus, students with physical disabilities are immediately ruled out. How then can this outcome meet the first assumption of applying to all students? An alternative outcome that includes the entire spectrum of unique physical characteristics would be "Demonstrates a sense of physical well-being."

In the Responsibility and Independence Domain, an outcome is "Demonstrates age appropriate independence." Again, the emphasis on age-appropriateness immediately rules out many children with significant developmental disabilities. Given the NCEO assumption that the outcome should apply to *all* children, we are interested in learning more about its rationale of how this outcome could possibly apply to preschoolers who experience significant delays in independent behavior.

Furthermore, we have major concerns about the cultural interpretations and again wonder how cultural diversity is respected throughout all of the outcomes. For example, one of the indicators related to age-appropriate independence is: "Percent of children who separate easily from parent/guardians in familiar and unfamiliar situations." That what is age-appropriate in a Latino culture may not be age-appropriate in an Anglo culture is reflected in the following:

> Juaaez (1985) related the importance of recognizing different norms around childrearing that exists for many Latino families as compared to Anglo families. In illustration, Latino families find it acceptable for preteens to sit on the mother's lap. Preschoolers who drink from a baby bottle may not be admonished. Moreover, it is normal in these families for members to sit close to one another and to have direct physical contact regardless of age. Anglo professionals might view this closeness as symbiotic behavior and as unacceptable. (Zuniga, 1992, p. 164)

In such situations, who determines age-appropriateness?

We note that NCEO is developing a guide for translating the indicators presented here into ones that are more individually based. This is a very positive step, but we believe that NCEO, educators, and families must be very cognizant to ensure that outcomes and indicators are not implemented in a way that restricts or separates students with disabilities and students from diverse cultural backgrounds because of their inability to meet norms generally expected by Anglo educators.

We would like to see stronger ties made between how the outcomes and indicators are stated and their rationale, and the "Guidelines for Appropriate Curriculum Content and Assessment" developed jointly by the National Association for the Education of Young Children (NAEYC) and the National Association of Early Childhood Specialists in State Departments of Education (NAECS/SDE). These guidelines, representing more than a decade of work defining best practice in early childhood, apply to children from 3-8 years old. They include twenty curriculum guidelines that we believe form an excellent basis for conceptualizing a philosophy for outcomes and indicators as well as the specification of outcomes and indicators. One of the guidelines addresses issues of normal/ age-appropriate expectations versus individual and culturally diverse expectations: "Curriculum goals are realistic and attainable for most children in the designated age range for which they were designed" (Bredekamp & Rosegrant, 1992). The explanatory material for this guideline states:

> Curriculum decisions about when children are expected to acquire knowledge and skills are based on age-group, individual, and cultural expectations. Curriculum expectations of young children are flexible and dynamic rather than deterministic and lock-step since there is no universal sequence of skills development. The curriculum allows for children to work at different levels on different activities and does not require all of the children to do the same thing at the same time. (Bredekamp & Rosegrant, 1992, p. 20)

Because several of the domains of the NCEO model are couched in normal development/age-appropriate expectations, we believe that there is the potential for confusion. We recommend that there be a philosophy statement that accompanies the outcomes and indicators and that the similarities and differences between the NCEO model and the "Guidelines for Appropriate Curriculum Content and Assessment" developed by NAEYC and NAECS/SDE be clearly specified. There is a danger that normal development/age-appropriate outcomes will have a deterministic impact on the curriculum.

The bottom line is that there should be a clear recognition of the importance of framing outcomes to respect the individual and culturally diverse characteristics of students. In an age of diversity, accountability measures must honor the fundamental premise of inclusion that "all children belong." We believe the outcomes related to normal development and age-appropriate expectations do not meet that litmus test.

FAMILY INVOLVEMENT OUTCOMES AND INDICATORS

In the introduction to this article, it is stated that stakeholders wanted the model to "reflect the importance of focusing on outcomes related to the involvement and support *of* the family and community." This is a laudable goal which we strongly support. We do note a major discontinuity, however, in the shift in emphasis from the support *of* the family to assessing the support *by* the family. Many of the indicators specified for the outcomes involve delicate judgments about the "appropriateness" of how parents assume their responsibilities. Examples of such indicators include the following:

- "Percent of children whose family system positively supports their development"
- "Percent of parents with appropriate parenting skills to anticipate and meet developmental needs of children."

Missing are family outcomes and indicators focusing on collaborative educational decision-making which would seem to be at the heart of effective home-school partnerships. It appears that these outcomes are written for the families rather than for the schools, with the onus on families to demonstrate their adequacy as parents, rather than on the schools to enhance, develop, and honor family participation. Such outcomes represent radical changes in the nature and responsibilities of early childhood educators.

By having outcomes and indicators for family performance, is it an implied commitment that the school will be offering comprehensive family support services? For example, given the indicator of: "Percent of families with adequate social and economic resources to appropriately parent children," will schools be providing these resources or will educators provide service coordination to assist families in finding these resources? If so, significant policy reform will be necessary to provide re-direction of funding streams as well as comprehensive changes in preservice and inservice education, and development of service integration of educational, health, mental health, and social services at the community level.

COMPOSITION OF STAKEHOLDERS

In reviewing the stakeholder list, we are unsure of the proportion of individuals with disabilities and parents of children with disabilities that were part of this stakeholder constituency. We also do not know the cultural diversity that was represented. We believe that constituency groups should be comprised of a substantial number of consumers (preferably 50%), and that diversity in terms of racial/ethnic background and socio-economic status should characterize the representation. We would like to recommend that NCEO's formal reports specify the consumer composition and cultural diversity represented by the stakeholders.

CONCLUSION

Our strongest endorsement of the NCEO approach is the inclusive and unitary orientation. We appreciate what it takes to formulate a new framework. Whatever criticisms and concerns we have are in the spirit of helping to shed some light on this new path, and we commend NCEO for its initial groundwork.

REFERENCES

Bredekamp, S., & Rosegrant, T. (1992). *Reaching potentials: Appropriate curriculum and assessment for young children* (Vol. 1). Washington, DC: National Association for the Education of Young Children.

Zuniga, M. E. (1992). In E. W. Lynch, & M. J. Hanson (Eds.), *Developing cross-cultural competence: A guide for working with young children and their families* (pp. 151-179). Baltimore, MD: Paul H. Brookes.

Future Directions in the Education of Students with Disabilities

Martha L. Thurlow
James E. Ysseldyke
Kristin M. Geenen

National Center on Educational Outcomes
University of Minnesota

SUMMARY. There are four main issues that will become the playing fields for future developments in educational outcomes for students with disabilities. These emerging issues are: implementation of Goals 2000, opportunity-to-learn standards, assessment accommodations, and accountability. The implications of these areas for identifying and promoting educational outcomes for students with disabilities are examined here, against the backdrop of the recent Educate America Act (Goals 2000). We begin with a discussion of the current buzz words associated with outcomes: Outcome-Based Education (OBE) and Outcome-Based Assessment (OBA). We conclude with some implications of the most current reform efforts for special and related services providers.

The development of this article was supported in part by a Cooperative Agreement (H159C00004) between the University of Minnesota and the U.S. Department of Education, Office of Special Education Programs. Points of view or opinions expressed in the article are not necessarily those of the department or offices within it.

Address correspondence to: Martha L. Thurlow, 350 Elliott Hall, 75 East River Road, University of Minnesota, Minneapolis, MN 55455.

[Haworth co-indexing entry note]: "Future Directions in the Education of Students with Disabilities." Thurlow, Martha L., James E. Ysseldyke, and Kristin M. Geenen. Co-published simultaneously in *Special Services in the Schools* (The Haworth Press, Inc.) Vol. 9, No. 2, 1994, pp. 193-208; and: *Educational Outcomes for Students with Disabilities* (ed: James E. Ysseldyke, and Martha L. Thurlow) The Haworth Press, Inc., 1994, pp. 193-208. Multiple copies of this article/chapter may be purchased from The Haworth Document Delivery Center [1-800-3-HAWORTH; 9:00 a.m. - 5:00 p.m. (EST)].

193

Growing dissatisfaction with America's schools has led to an era of educational reform. As part of the reform movement, educators are engaged in documenting the products of America's educational system as a starting point for improving them. Current school reform can be characterized not only by a shift in focus from the process to the outcomes of education, but also by an increase in the involvement of larger political systems. Educational reform is no longer the sole responsibility of local schools; rather, our nation's governors, business leaders and even presidents are participating (McLaughlin, Schofield, & Warren, in press). Yet, there has been little discussion about how students with disabilities will be included in this broad attempt to restructure education (McLaughlin et al., in press). The future directions of educational outcomes for students with disabilities will be guided by this larger reform effort, and specifically by the implementation of Goals 2000, opportunity-to-learn standards, assessment accommodations, and accountability. Significant activity, some of which was spurred by the Educate America Act (Goals 2000), is occurring around these issues.

OUTCOME-BASED EDUCATION

Outcome-based education (OBE) may be the first term that comes to mind for many involved in debates and discussions about America's education. Gearing educational programs to focus on pre-selected outcomes is not a new concept, particularly to special educators, who have set goals and objectives for students since P.L. 94-142. However, OBE has received considerable attention lately because some schools, districts and states have implemented OBE for *all* their students. The original intention of OBE was to design a curriculum that ensured that all students would gain mastery in prescribed outcome areas. Instruction was to be modified to accommodate the time needed by individual students to reach these outcomes. Thus, a direct link would be established between instruction, assessment, and the targeted outcomes of the educational process. These outcomes included educational results such as: collaboration skills, self-direction in learning, complex thinking, respect for self worth and respect for individual differences. Here the quagmire surrounding OBE begins. Many states attempting to implement OBE met with opposition from those who argued that the teaching of values was inappropriately seeping into the public schools. Heated debates followed, and the debates fanned the flames of belief that OBE stressed values more than academic content.

As groups became more vocal, additional objections to OBE were raised, including charges that OBE "dummys down" the curriculum. The thrust of this argument is that OBE sacrifices academic quality for mediocrity, resulting in penalizing gifted students (Smetanka, 1993). The basis for this concern may be a confusion of OBE with mastery learning, an educational approach that previously was rejected for its emphasis on basic skills rather than higher order abilities (Olson, 1993).

Another criticism of OBE is that the goals and standards are often ill-defined. Too much jargon accompanies OBE curricula, and educators find it difficult to teach and assess student progress toward ambiguous outcomes such as "the student will be a community contributor." An additional source of resistance to OBE is typical of any reform effort–fear of change and the change process. One parent who pulled her son out of a high school that had adopted OBE said: "I don't want my kids experimented on while teachers try to figure out what's going on" (Smetanka, 1993).

A few schools and states have attempted to circumvent the controversy associated with OBE by avoiding the term "outcomes." Terms such as "results-oriented education" or "quality education," have been used instead. (For more information on OBE see Ysseldyke and Thurlow and Massanari, in this volume.)

OUTCOME-BASED ASSESSMENT

Outcome-based assessments (OBA) often accompany OBE curricula. Outcome-based assessments are designed to measure a student's progress toward achieving an outcome targeted by the curriculum and instruction. Due to the increasing popularity of cooperative learning and other less traditional approaches to curriculum and instruction, greater emphasis has been given to complex skills. Since the goal of OBE is to keep a direct link between curriculum, instruction, and assessment, OBA must reflect the higher order skills taught in the classrooms. Thus, outcomes, and subsequently assessments, increasingly target higher-order skills such as problem solving, synthesis, observations and creativity.

Traditional assessments (norm referenced, multiple choice) stress repetition of facts or test-taking skills rather than measuring more complex skills. Traditional tests tend to report the relative standing of students rather than their demonstration of mastery. Furthermore, traditional assessments focus on breadth rather than depth, running the risk of testing concepts to which students have not received exposure. The function of OBA (to strengthen the link between instruction and assessment and to test for mastery) encourages alternatives to traditional assessment. One alternative is to require students to construct rather than select (multiple choice) their responses. This method is more likely to test higher-order skills and is more typical of real-life demands. OBA often incorporates "performance" (constructing an answer) and "authentic" (real-life problems) assessment procedures in an attempt to sample student progress toward the outcomes designated by the OBE curriculum.

Many of the future activities in determining educational outcomes for students with disabilities will include OBA. Currently, many of the characteristics of OBA parallel existing special education assessment procedures. Students' IEPs document the link between curriculum and instruction, and assessment. These linkages are one goal of OBA. A second characteristic of OBA is an emphasis on performance assessment and/or authentic assessment. Special education has a long history of assessing students skills via performance on authentic tasks, particularly in the assessment of students with severe disabilities or sensory impairments (Coutinho & Malouf, 1993). Thus, OBA may provide a greater opportunity for assessing the knowledge and skills of students with disabilities in conjunction with regular education students. This may, in turn, result in greater congruence between instruction, curriculum and outcomes in special and general education.

GOALS 2000 AND STANDARDS

The purpose of P.L. 103-227 (Goals 2000: Educate America Act) is to "provide a framework for meeting the National Education Goals" (U.S. Congress, 1993, Sec. 2). This legislation provides not only a vision of excellence for America's educational system, but also offers support in the form of grants, consortia, and certifying groups to assist state and local school reform efforts. Specifically, Goals 2000 sets the agenda for U.S. education reform by establishing the nation's goals for education, the continued monitoring of progress toward the goals by the National Education Goals Panel (NEGP), the setting of standards, and the formation of a National Education Standards and Improvement Council (NESIC) to certify and approve standards and assessments. Yet, the most significant component of the Educate America Act may be the law's commitment to including students with disabilities within national reform. In Section 3(1) it is stated that:

> the terms "all students" and "all children" mean students or children from a broad range of backgrounds and circumstances, including . . . students or children with disabilities. (U.S. Congress, 1993)

Thus, for the first time, federal legislation that does not specifically target special education programs explicitly requires the consideration of students with disabilities in programs that will affect all students. In some sections, specific requirements are outlined to assure that the policy of including all students translates into practice. A few examples of Goals 2000's attention to incorporating policy that targets the educational outcomes of students with disabilities are listed in Table 1. These quotes clearly illustrate an emphasis on funding programs that specify how students with disabilities will be accommodated.

The slogan attached to Goals 2000, "National Standards, Local Reforms" highlights the responsibility of state and local education agencies to develop or choose programs that include students with disabilities. Here, a number of issues regarding students with disabilities emerge. In particular, Goals 2000 refers to the development of standards for all students, leaving states and local districts to wrestle with decisions such as: (a) are separate standards needed for students with disabilities? (b) who decides which standards apply to which students? (c) if a range of performance is expected, what is an acceptable range? (d) what will be the critical keys to implementing the goals, standards, and assessments in a way that includes all

TABLE 1. Selected References to Students with Disabilities in Goals 2000

"To the extent feasible, the membership of the Council (NESIC) shall be geographically representative of the United States and reflect the diversity of the United States with regard to . . . disability characteristic" 212(c)(2).

"Not less than one-third of the individuals nominated and appointed . . . shall have expertise or background in the educational needs of children who . . . have disabilities" 212(c)(3).

Opportunity to learn standards will address "the capability of teachers to provide high-quality instruction to meet diverse learning needs in each content area to all students" 213(c)(2)(B).

"The Council shall certify State assessments only if such assessments include all students and provide for the adaptations and accommodations necessary to permit the participation of all students with diverse learning needs" 213(f)(2)(F).

Development of the assessments identified by the State School Improvement Plan must "provide for the participation in such assessments of all students with diverse learning needs" 306(c)(1)(B)(III).

The peer review process of State's improvement plan "shall be representative of the diversity of the United States with regard to . . . disability characteristics" 306(n)(1).

After the first year, State School Improvement Plans shall "use the remainder of such assistance for State activities . . . such as—providing special attention to the needs of . . . disabled . . . students" 308(b)(2)(D).

---

students? The language of Goals 2000 is very clear; the educational outcomes of students with disabilities are to be considered in the standards-setting effort. Yet, some suggest that standards designed so that all students have the potential to achieve them, will result in lowering standards to the level of minimum competencies. Most educators and policymakers believe we should avoid the reduction of standards to minimum competencies. Few are willing to recreate the dissatisfying results of minimum competency testing. But, the premise behind standards–high expectations for performance will increase the likelihood that students will attain high levels of achievement–may only be obtained by identifying a range of acceptable performance or designating different standards for various groups of students. A critical component to resolving this issue will be to adopt student outcome areas that represent goals for all students, such as high school completion and literacy. The knowledge and skill standards for each goal area may be allowed to vary or contain a range of acceptable performance levels. The key challenge is to resolve this issue while retaining high expectations for all students.

Additional issues raised by Goals 2000 will affect future developments in educational outcomes for students with disabilities. These issues relate to translating opportunity to learn and assessment accommodation policy into practice. Both of these are addressed in the next sections of this paper. Regardless of how these issues are resolved, for better or for worse, it is important to realize that the commitment of Goals 2000 to improving the educational outcomes of students with disabilities, alongside those of general education students, is a blueprint for future federal Department of Education programs (Sklaroff, 1994).

ASSESSMENT ACCOMMODATIONS

Too often, students with disabilities are being excluded from large-scale traditional and alternative ("authentic," performance) assessments. Yet, these assessment programs are frequently the cornerstone of reform programs such as OBE, Goals 2000, and accountability. The results of this practice may be that students with disabilities do not fully benefit from these reform efforts.

The current focus on assessment is in response to the realization that standardizing, monitoring and evaluating the process of education does not guarantee positive student outcomes. In short, we do not really know what works the best for all students. Thus, policymakers can sidestep "having to spell out the ingredients of educational success" by emphasizing "outcomes" as the best indication that the educational process is meeting the needs of all students (Monk, 1992). Students with disabilities participate in many assessments, but most focus on matching student learning needs to eligibility criteria. This type of individualized assessment does not inform educators, policymakers, or other stakeholders about the progress of these students toward our national goals. Rather, large scale assessment programs, such as the National Assessment of Educational Progress (NAEP), document student progress toward national goals and standards. Currently, NAEP includes only half of all students with disabilities, and there is wide variation in the inclusion rate among individual states (33% to 87%) (McGrew, Thurlow, Shriner, & Spiegel, 1992). Thus state comparisons are difficult to make and we do not really know whether the outcomes of students with disabilities are being improved by the national education agenda. Furthermore, excluding students with disabilities from large-scale accountability assessments results in ranking some students as more important than others (Ysseldyke, Thurlow, & Geenen, 1994). A strong commitment to holding educational systems accountable for the outcomes of all students requires the inclusion of the performance of students with disabilities in accountability assessments and reports. These reports are often the basis for many policy decisions.

Students with disabilities are excluded from large-scale assessment programs for several reasons. High stakes assessments involve consequences such as: student graduation, staff wage increases, funding for programs, and schools' public recognition (school choice); in some cases the very existence of a job or entire school may be contingent on demonstrating results. Thus, some schools or staff hold the attitude that including students with disabilities in testing is risky. Furthermore, the decision about which students to include is often deferred to the IEP team, resulting in great variability in the criteria for inclusion in accountability assessments. Some argue that a national set of inclusion guidelines needs to replace the diverse array of state and local guidelines that currently exist. Resolving this issue will have significant implications for the outcomes of students with disabilities. If established, national guidelines for inclusion may follow the precedent that Kentucky has established. All students with disabilities are expected to participate in some part of the Kentucky Instructional Results Information System (KIRIS), with or without accommodations (Ysseldyke et al., 1994).

The second major reason for excluding students with disabilities is a resistance to providing accommodations. The five major types of accommodations are: (a) Presentation format: Braille, large-print, oral or signing delivery of directions, and interpretation of directions; (b) Response format: template or point to response; provide response orally or in sign language or by typewriter or computer; (c) Setting of test: alone in carrel, small group, at home, in special education class; (d) Timing of test: extended time, more breaks, extending sessions over several days; (e) Other approaches, such as out of level testing (Thurlow, Ysseldyke, & Silverstein, 1993). Large scale assessments, such as NAEP, do not have a history of allowing accommodations in assessments. At the state and local levels, students with disabilities may be denied these accommodations because the staff decides the accommodations are too difficult to provide (expensive, personnel time, etc.), or they are viewed as a threat to the test's psychometric soundness. The uncertainty surrounding acceptable accommodations to standardized testing procedures results from a lack of knowledge about the effects of various modifications on the reliability and validity of the results. The guidelines provided by state departments on assessment accommodations vary greatly in detail (from one sentence to 72 pages) and content (what one state recommends, another prohibits) (Thurlow et al., 1993). One solution to collecting intelligible, comparable, and valid data on all students may be to analyze and report the data separately by accommodation (Ysseldyke & Thurlow, 1993).

Regardless of the difficulties associated with providing accommodations in testing, federal law clearly supports their use. For example, excluding students with disabilities from accountability assessments that directly impact policy decisions may violate the 14th Amendment, which guarantees the right to equal educational opportunities and requires due process when state laws adversely affect an individual. The Americans with Disabilities Act requires businesses that receive federal funds and licensing boards to make all exams accessible to individuals with disabilities. In order to receive funding from the Goals 2000 $105 million in grants, states are required to design "State assessments that include all students and provide for the adaptations and accommodations necessary to permit the participation of all students with diverse learning needs" (Goals 2000 (213(f)(2)(F)). One issue emerging from this legislation is whether current law (ADA, Goals 2000) requires that accommodations be provided regardless of the purpose (or stakes) of the test or the disability.

A related issue is the lack of educational policies or testing publishers that offer guidelines for determining which accommodations are appropriate for individual students. Determining when and which accommodations are appropriate will be of great concern in the near future.

Two additional concerns are raised in the inclusion and accommodation of students with disabilities in testing: (a) Does testing cause unnecessary stress for students with disabilities? and (b) What tests should be administered to students in ungraded classrooms? Alternative assessments, such as portfolio assessments, may offer a solution to these troubling questions. Portfolios collect the best work of each student. They may be more laborious to assess, but students are afforded the opportunity to demonstrate their abilities and provide input into future education reform. This is one reason that Kentucky moved toward emphasizing the portfolio portion of their accountability program (Ysseldyke, Thurlow, & Geenen, 1994).

OPPORTUNITY-TO-LEARN STANDARDS

Goals 2000 requires states to set content and performance standards for all students, including those with diverse learning needs. Yet, the responsibility for ensuring that students reach content and performance standards falls squarely on the educational system. The opportunity-to-learn standards proposed in Goals 2000 demand that every effort be made to develop in all students the knowledge and skills identified by the standards. Thus, Goals 2000 acknowledges that expecting more from students must be accompanied by providing them with the opportunity to learn what is expected and tested. The most influential tenet of this policy is the definition of "opportunity to learn." Though ill-defined within Goals 2000, opportunity-to-learn standards clearly emphasize more than exposure to a curriculum. Section 213(c)(2)(B) states that "opportunity-to-learn standards will address the capabilities of teachers to meet diverse learning needs in each content area" This call for equity in terms of meeting individual learning needs does not assist in clarifying the definition and documentation of opportunity to learn. There are conflicting opinions on what determines opportunity to learn. It may include amount of funding or other resources, time in class, content coverage, quality of instructional practices, or academic engaged time. Depending on which definition is adopted, various issues related to outcomes of education for students with disabilities will emerge. Specifically, these decisions must be made: (a) Should we define opportunity to learn differently for students with disabilities? (b) Do we hold out for equal time or equal opportunity, and if we assume that all students will be held to the same or similar standards, how do we identify the obstacles that are hindering the student's progress? (For a more detailed analysis of opportunity-to-learn standards and implications for students with disabilities, see Ysseldyke, Thurlow, & Shin this volume.)

Currently, there is opposition to the idea of opportunity-to-learn standards. This opposition arises from the complexity of the issue and concern that opportunity-to-learn standards will usurp local control and increase federal involvement. Furthermore, some local schools are anxious to avoid lawsuits by parents who claim the school failed to meet the standard ("Special Report," 1994). Schools may choose not to submit standards to NESIC. However, failure to participate in the Goals 2000 grant program will not make opportunity-to-learn standards disappear. In fact Congress may require schools to document opportunity to learn in order to receive funding from the billion dollar Chapter 1 program.

ACCOUNTABILITY

Accountability programs, like opportunity-to-learn standards, attempt to insure the provision of instruction and curriculum in which students can and do learn. The distinction between the two programs is that opportunity to learn stresses the processes of education (exposure to curriculum, teachers' ability to meet the needs of diverse learners, etc.) and accountability focuses on the product of education. Accountability programs may also include holding larger systems (building, district or state) responsible for providing a quality education as documented by student outcomes. Accountability may be defined as "a systematic method to assure those inside and outside the educational system that schools and students are moving toward desired goals" (Center for Policy Options, 1994, p. 2). Accountability programs typically include consequences for the system's performance. The consequences are administered on the basis of student achievement of the desired outcomes, and may include some combination of reward and sanctions, and/or public recognition (Ysseldyke et al., 1994).

Reward and sanction systems typically involve state distribution of incentives or penalties to students, teachers, principals, and even superintendents for poor or favorable accountability results. The incentives may include: monetary awards to teachers, schools, or districts; accreditation of program or school; increased technical assistance; waivers or regulatory flexibility. Penalties for poor performance may include: failure to graduate, loss of funding, mandated corrective action, school closure or take-overs, or loss of personnel wages or jobs. Many of these consequences are considered "high-stakes," and are associated with unintended negative consequences for the outcomes of students with disabilities. For example, some states and districts that made teacher wage increases contingent upon student performance found teachers to become less supportive of integrating students with disabilities into their classroom. A few teachers have even encouraged low performing students to stay home on testing days. Educational outcomes for students with disabilities will be affected by the intensity and level (individual or system) of accountability consequences.

The exclusion of students with disabilities may be discouraged by a public disclosure system that reports the participation rates of these students in the accountability assessment. Typically, accountability systems produce school, district, or state report cards that document the educational systems' effectiveness. Based on comparisons to other schools or districts, educational systems are rewarded through public recognition, accreditation, or parental choice programs for good performance. Including *all* students in the accountability assessment, documentation, and reporting programs is critical to the validity of these comparisons.

Resistance to including students with disabilities stems from the separation of special and general education. Special education is viewed by some as the primary source of responsibility for the educational outcomes of students with disabilities. Yet increasingly, regular education is providing the context for special education students' learning. Furthermore, special education accountability programs are based on monitoring for compliance and the presence of a student in a program (i.e., child count). Neither method indicates whether students are achieving desired results. Recently, the New York City school system was attacked for its lack of accountability in Special Education programs. Critics noted that the only available information on New York special education students is that spending for special education students is twice the amount per child of general education, yet the outcomes for special education students appear to be worse (e.g., the city's 14 most 'violent' schools are all devoted to special education) (Miller, 1994).

There will be increasing demands for alternative ways to account for the outcomes of students with disabilities. For example, Goals 2000 State Improvement Plans will encourage educators to account for the results of special education. State Improvement Plans are required to contain strategies for improving accountability ((306)(e)). The Goals 2000 accountability requirement specifically excludes high stakes consequences. Thus, students with disabilities may be more likely to participate. Furthermore, by the second year, the State Improvement Plans must devote special attention to meeting the needs of students with disabilities ((308)(b)(2)(D)). It will be interesting to observe how states meet these accountability requirements. As states receive these education-reform planning grants, more states will be looking for ways to demonstrate accountability in special education.

Accountability for other federally funded programs is currently mandated. Title 1 (previously Chapter 1) continues to require evaluations of student performance in order to hold systems accountable for student progress. In general, accountability programs have increased in popularity. In a recent *Education Week* article, Richardson (1994) wrote that linking rewards to school restructuring or improvement of student achievement has become more popular in the past 10 years; half of the states are funding some type of incentive program. As the prevalence of accountability programs increases, so will the discussion on making educational accountability decisions for students with disabilities. Issues that must be addressed in demonstrating that education works for students with disabilities include: (a) Will holding systems accountable for the results of their programs for students with disabilities encourage a greater effort to create the conditions that support these outcomes? (b) Will punitive consequences for poor performance result in more effective interventions? (c) What is the most appropriate level of accountability–student, teacher, principal, school, district or state? (d) If students are held accountable (i.e., graduation contingent upon demonstration of mastery), how will accommodations be made for students with disabilities? (e) What type of data demonstrates that education works for students with disabilities?

A STUDY

By October 1994 a study will be initiated that will have an impact on the direction of emerging developments in educational outcomes for students with disabilities. Section 1015 of Goals 2000 designates $600,000 for conducting a "comprehensive study of the inclusion of children with disabilities in school reform activities" assisted under this law. The study is to address many of the issues outlined in this article, including: standards, assessment accommodations, and accountability. In addition, the study is required to examine the relationship of the Goals 2000: Educate America Act to other Federal Laws (IDEA) that affect special education. There is a provision for addressing any other issues deemed relevant. The results of the study will be presented within two years of its start-up. By mandating this study, the Federal government expresses a strong commitment to including students with disabilities in school reform.

CONCLUSION

For the first time, policymakers are attempting to raise the educational achievements of *all* American students. Previously, legislation has singled-out students with disabilities in an effort to protect their rights to an equitable education. Current reform policy now looks to improve the outcomes of all students. Thus, Goals 2000, opportunity to learn and accountability are not general nor special education programs. They are designed to assist *all* students in regaining America's global competitiveness.

For many, it will be difficult to understand the need to examine these larger educational contexts and where students with special needs fit into the context. As discussion of the issues outlined in this paper grows, professionals who provide special and related services to students with disabilities will become more involved. Much discussion has focused on integrating students with disabilities into the classroom, but future issues will involve the inclusion of these students in the larger educational restructuring programs. Goals 2000 and other reform efforts will create a demand for input from special services providers on how best to implement Goals 2000, develop opportunity-to-learn standards, design and maintain accountability programs, and provide assessment accommodations. Input from special educators, school psychologists, occupational and physical therapists, and speech and language specialists is critical to designing policies and programs that maximally include and benefit students with disabilities. At the classroom level, one "trickle down effect" of national and state policies may be the alignment of IEP goals, special education instruction and curriculum to state and national standards. Special education students may find themselves participating in more state assessments in new and interesting ways. In the near future, parents of special education students may be surprised to see their child's results included in state and local report cards.

In a more general sense, educators will need to ask themselves: What do my students know? What can they do? What should they know and be able to do? How does this fit with my nation's or state's goals? How do I create the learning environment that will get them there? It is hoped that this mind-set will be the result of the current policy of reform and will translate into services that allow *all* students to meet the national goals by the year 2000.

REFERENCES

Coutinho, M., & Malouf, D. (1993). Performance assessment and children with disabilities: Issues and possibilities. *Teaching Exceptional Children, 25*(4), 63-67.

Center for Policy Options. (1994). *Issues & options in outcomes-based accountability for students with disabilities.* College Park, MD: University of Maryland.

McGrew, K. S., Thurlow, M. L., Shriner, J. G., & Spiegel, A. N. (1992). *Inclusion of students with disabilities in national and state data collection programs* (Technical Report 2). Minneapolis, MN: National Center on Educational Outcomes.

McLaughlin, M. J., Schofield, P. F., & Warren, S. H. (in press). Educational reform: Issues for the inclusion of students with disabilities. In M. Coutinho & A. Repp (Eds.), *Enhancing the integration of children with disabilities.* Baltimore: Brookes/Cole.

Miller, L. (1994, July 13). Lack of accountability in special education program blasted. *Education Week,* p. 5.

Monk, D. (1992). Education productivity research: An update and assessment of its role in education finance reform. *Educational Evaluation and Policy Analysis, 14*(4), 307-332.

Olson, L. (1993, December 15). Who's afraid of OBE? *Education Week,* p. 25.

Richardson, J. (1994, June 8). Incentive plans, once controversial, now common. *Education Week,* p. 17.

Sklaroff, S. (1994, April 20). Goals 2000 seen spurring 'inclusion' movement. *Education Week,* p. 5.

Smetanka, M. J. (1993, September 12). Outcome-based education faces critical questions. *Minneapolis Star Tribune,* p. 18A.

Special report on opportunity-to-learn standards. (1994, March 23). *Education Week,* p. 33.

Thurlow, M. L., Ysseldyke, J. E., & Silverstein, B. (1994). *Testing accommodations for students with disabilities: A review of the literature* (Synthesis Report 4). Minneapolis, MN: National Center on Educational Outcomes.

U.S. Congress. (1993, March). *Goals 2000: Educate America Act. Public Law 103-227.* 103d Congress.

Ysseldyke, J., & Thurlow, M. (1993). *Views on inclusion and testing accommodations for students with disabilities* (Synthesis Report 7). Minneapolis, MN: National Center on Educational Outcomes.

Ysseldyke, J., Thurlow, M., & Geenen, K. (1994). *Implementation of alternative methods for making educational accountability decisions for students with disabilities.* Minneapolis, MN: National Center on Educational Outcomes.

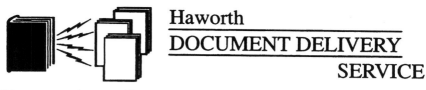

Haworth
DOCUMENT DELIVERY
SERVICE

This new service provides a single-article order form for any article from a Haworth journal.

- *Time Saving:* No running around from library to library to find a specific article.
- *Cost Effective:* All costs are kept down to a minimum.
- *Fast Delivery:* Choose from several options, including same-day FAX.
- *No Copyright Hassles:* You will be supplied by the original publisher.
- *Easy Payment:* Choose from several easy payment methods.

Open Accounts Welcome for . . .
- Library Interlibrary Loan Departments
- Library Network/Consortia Wishing to Provide Single-Article Services
- Indexing/Abstracting Services with Single Article Provision Services
- Document Provision Brokers and Freelance Information Service Providers

---

MAIL or *FAX* THIS ENTIRE ORDER FORM TO:

Haworth Document Delivery Service The Haworth Press, Inc. 10 Alice Street Binghamton, NY 13904-1580	**or FAX:** (607) 722-6362 **or CALL:** 1-800-3-HAWORTH (1-800-342-9678; 9am-5pm EST)

PLEASE SEND ME PHOTOCOPIES OF THE FOLLOWING SINGLE ARTICLES:

1) Journal Title: _____

    Vol/Issue/Year: _____ Starting & Ending Pages: _____

Article Title: _____

_____

2) Journal Title: _____

    Vol/Issue/Year: _____ Starting & Ending Pages: _____

Article Title: _____

_____

3) Journal Title: _____

    Vol/Issue/Year: _____ Starting & Ending Pages: _____

Article Title: _____

_____

4) Journal Title: _____

    Vol/Issue/Year: _____ Starting & Ending Pages: _____

Article Title: _____

_____

(See other side for Costs and Payment Information)

COSTS: Please figure your cost to order quality copies of an article.
1. Set-up charge per article: $8.00
          ($8.00 × number of separate articles)   _____
2. Photocopying charge for each article:
               1-10 pages: $1.00   _____

               11-19 pages: $3.00   _____

               20-29 pages: $5.00   _____

               30+ pages: $2.00/10 pages   _____

3. Flexicover (optional): $2.00/article   _____
4. Postage & Handling: US: $1.00 for the first article/
               $.50 each additional article   _____

               Federal Express: $25.00   _____

               Outside US: $2.00 for first article/
               $.50 each additional article _____
5. Same-day FAX service: $.35 per page   _____

GRAND TOTAL: _____

METHOD OF PAYMENT: (please check one)
❑ Check enclosed   ❑ Please ship and bill. PO # _____
          (sorry we can ship and bill to bookstores only! All others must pre-pay)
❑ Charge to my credit card: ❑ Visa; ❑ MasterCard; ❑ American Express;

Account Number:_____ Expiration date:_____

Signature: ✗_____

Name: _____ Institution: _____

Address: _____

_____

City: _____ State:_____ Zip:_____

Phone Number: _____ FAX Number: _____

MAIL or *FAX* THIS ENTIRE ORDER FORM TO:

Haworth Document Delivery Service	**or FAX:** (607) 722-6362
The Haworth Press, Inc.	**or CALL:** 1-800-3-HAWORTH
10 Alice Street	(1-800-342-9678; 9am-5pm EST)
Binghamton, NY 13904-1580	